Heartbreak and Heart Disease

Heartbreak and Heart Disease

A MIND/BODY PRESCRIPTION FOR
HEALING THE HEART

Stephen T. Sinatra, M.D.

FOREWORD BY
ROSEMARY ELLEN GUILEY

KEATS PUBLISHING, INC. NEW CANAAN, CONNECTICUT

Heartbreak and Heart Disease is not intended as medical advice. Its intention is solely informational and educational. Please consult a medical or health professional should the need for one be indicated. The information in this book lends itself to self-help. For obvious reasons, the author and publisher cannot take the medical or legal responsibility of having the contents herein considered as a prescription for everyone. Either you, or the physician who examines and treats you, must take the responsibility for the uses of this book.

Library of Congress Cataloging-in-Publication Data

Sinatra, Stephen T.
    Heartbreak and heart disease / Stephen T. Sinatra
       p.   cm.
    Includes bibliographical references and index
    ISBN 0-87983-974-0
    1. Heart—Diseases—Psychosomatic aspects. I. Title
RC682.S49   1996
616.1'2'0019—dc20   96-23066
                                          CIP

HEARTBREAK AND HEART DISEASE

Published by Keats, a division of NTC/Contemporary Publishing Group, Inc.
4255 West Touhy Avenue, Lincolnwood, Illinois 60646-1975 U.S.A.

Copyright © 1996, 1999 by Stephen T. Sinatra, M.D.

Printed and bound in the United States of America
International Standard Book Number: 0-87983-974-0
10 9 8 7 6 5 4 3 2 1

Dedication

———— ✑ ————

To the late John Bellis, M.D., psychiatrist and bioenergetic therapist, trusted colleague and friend, who succumbed to heart disease in March, 1995. John's presence touched many lives as a poet, writer, analyst and physician. His love, comfort, and words of wisdom after my father's death helped me through a most difficult time in my life. His spirit lives on through this book as he was instrumental in editing some of the material prior to his illness. It was John's inspiration that was pivotal in helping me complete this long overdue project.

And to all my patients who have shared their struggles and deepest secrets with me.

Acknowledgments

———— 🦢 ————

The research and writing of this book took at least a decade to accomplish. I am especially indebted to Dr. Alexander Lowen, my bioenergetic teacher who placed me on the path to write this book beginning in 1985.

To Meyer Friedman, M.D., the pioneer on personality, behavior and heart disease: your work became my life's passion. To Robert Eliot, M.D., F.A.C.C.: I have always been indebted to your research on emotional stress and the heart.

To my cardiological colleagues who believe in the mind/body connection: Harvey Zarren, M.D., Richard Delaney, M.D., Bruno Cortis, M.D., Steven Horowitz, M.D., and Steven Kunkes, M.D.

To John Bustelos, CEO, Griffin Hospital, an innovator in complementary cardiology: your leading-edge programs on alternative cardiological care are, perhaps, the best in the country.

To Brendan Montano, M.D. and Holly Hatch, M.S.W., my good friends and colleagues who asked me to join them in their stress and illness workshops during the late 70's and early 80's. It was this interest that ignited my passion to become a bioenergetic therapist.

To all my trainers and therapists in my 10-year training program of bioenergetic analysis, I thank you all. A special thank you goes to Philip Helfaer, Ph.D. my trainer and mentor.

To Frank Hladky, Ph.D., Virginia Wink Hilton, Ph.D., Robert Hilton, Ph.D., Joyce Bellis and the late John Bellis,

M.D., John Pierrakos, M.D., Ben Shapiro, Ph.D., David Boadella, Ph.D., Vivian Guze and Hazel Stanley, Leslie Case, Ph.D., June Gray, Ph.D., David Campbell, M.B., Ed Svasta, M.S.W., Robert Lewis, M.D., Jes Jacobs, Angela Klopstech and Ellen Green: you have all been inspirational teachers and psychotherapists that I truly admire and respect.

To my loyal and very special office staff, thank you Rosemary Pontillo, Carol Gustamachio, Rebecca Rossick, Caron Maker and JoAnne Rena.

To Sun King Wan, M.D. and Laurel Gay, P.A.-C., my cardiological associates who took on the burden of additional clinical work as I was writing this book. I offer you my love and gratitude.

To Donna Chaput and Matt Dugan who assisted in endless hours typing the manuscript.

To Phyllis Herman, my editor at Keats Publishing: I thank you for your editing, guidance and direction. It was your enthusiasm and support that made this book a reality.

To Marilyn Anderson, M.A., Jerry Ainsworth, Ph.D., and Nicholas Palermo, D.O. for your heartfelt support.

To the "editorial team" at Phillips Publishing including Robert King, Julia B. Noble, Amy Painter, Karen Phillips, Karen Berney, and Roberta J. Lieberman: I thank you for *HeartSense.*

To Susan Graham, L.P.N. and massage therapist: I thank you for all your creativity, writing and editing. Your incredible knowledge about the "dark side" and how instrumental it is in healing has been a profound addition to this book. Your assistance in helping me write this chapter was much appreciated.

To JoAnne Piazza: your continued support for me over the years has touched my heart in so many ways. I treasure your loyality. Thank you for all the "heart" you have put into this book.

To my ex-wife, Susy Sinatra, my lifelong friend and mother

of my children who always gave me support during my early years as a doctor.

To my first family—my mother, E. Patricia Sinatra, my deceased father Charles Sinatra, my sisters Pam and Maria and my brother Richard: I have been so blessed with your presence in my life. To my second family—my children, March, Step and Drew: I offer you my unconditional love forever.

To Jan DeMarco, R.N., M.S.N., the woman in my life and my partner: you have been so understanding and supportive. I thank you for your editing, writing and all the times you nurtured me during the endless time it took to prepare this manuscript.

Contents

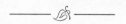

Foreword

———— 🖋 ————

Sensitivity is something we always hope to receive from a physician, but often it gets lost in the shuffle of crowded appointment books, charts, analyses of symptoms and tests. When I first met Dr. Stephen Sinatra, it was evident that sensitivity was high on his list of priorities. He is a doctor who truly walks a path with heart and soul—someone who has a deep understanding of the needs, longings and experiences of the human heart, and how those factors affect our health.

Dr. Sinatra was fortunate to see the importance of emotional and spiritual needs—the heart connection—early in his career. He saw how emotional losses, disappointments and stresses can literally create a state of heartbreak that can result in coronary artery disease—the leading cause of death in the industrialized world. We all suffer heartbreak during our lives. Dr. Sinatra's experiences coming to terms with his own heartbreak are frankly recounted in this book, as are the experiences of numerous patients.

When I read *Heartbreak and Heart Disease*, I resonated deeply with its message. In recent years, my interest in complementary healing has led me to develop my own ability in energy healing by taking instruction in various techniques. As I learned how to sense a person's energy field, I was astonished at the information that jumped forward. Not only do physical problems show up as disturbances in the energy field, but so do *emotional* issues—the scars and hurts we accumulate over time. The emotional issues point to root causes of physical problems.

I see many cases of the wounded and broken heart described in these pages by Dr. Sinatra. It is not uncommon to sense emotional wounds that are quite old. In fact, hurts that we think are long healed can remain deeply buried, leaking emotional toxins that continue to undermine our health. I encounter the wounded and broken heart so often that it seems that most of us unwittingly are the walking wounded, marching about with smiles on our faces but serious injuries in the centers of our being.

That is why the wisdom that Dr. Sinatra shares is so important. In approaching our health, we must pay attention to all facets of the beautiful diamond that is the total self.

Heartbreak and Heart Disease is a life-changing book, written in a warm and personal style by a physician who makes a sincere heart-to-heart connection with those he serves. *Heartbreak & Heart Disease* will change your approach to controllable factors concerning heart disease, such as diet and stress management. But there is more to a healthy heart than these. Dr. Sinatra pays special attention to the emotional "hidden" risk factors which manifest as behaviors and physiological conditions that can place one at risk for heart disease. Such hidden factors are often overlooked in mainstream health care.

Heartbreak and Heart Disease will help you uncover these hidden factors and take action. It will change the way you regard yourself and express your emotions. It will change the way you work and play, and the way you relate to others. It will even change the way you breathe.

A healthy heart and holistic living go hand in hand. When we are whole, everything in life blooms at full flower.

—Rosemary Ellen Guiley
Author, *The Miracle of Prayer* and
Blessings: Prayers for the Home and Family

Preface

Paul "Bear" Bryant, the "winningest" coach in college football, died suddenly of a massive heart attack just weeks following his retirement. Sadly, he joined the thousands of individuals who, after the loss of a vital connection or motivating force in their life, such as a spouse or a career, succumb to death. Coach Bryant was a "sudden death" victim. Research has shown that up to 50 percent of the time sudden death can be the first symptom of heart disease.

Underneath these cold, hard statistics emerges an equally important factor in the sudden death syndrome. This is the powerful, scientifically proven relationship between the mind and body. I believe Coach Bryant was one of the thousands of individuals who after experiencing a significant loss of relationship, of work, of meaning, or of hope lost his own life. Thus, the ineluctable link between heartbreak and heart disease—my focus throughout this book.

What is heartbreak? I define heartbreak as the emotional response to the loss of love and intimacy in life. Many cases on record attest to heartbreak being directly responsible for heart disease. In poetry, the heart and mind have always been considered interconnected, but until recently, medical science did not pay much attention to the relationship between the two. Increasingly, however, some cardiologists speak not only of angina, arrhythmia, or heart attack, but also of heartache resulting from the loss of vital connections. Such emotions can eventually lead to heartbreak or the literal breaking down of heart function.

Exploring the health effects of love and intimacy generates the following important questions:

- To what extent do emotional factors and one's own intrinsic personality play a part in heart disease?
- Are suppressed feelings and emotions significant?
- Do negative feelings such as abandonment, heartbreak, betrayal or humiliation create conditions that invite death?
- What part do positive emotions such as love, faith and good humor play in the process of healing and staying well?
- What is the significance of the way we breathe?

This book explores the power of the mind and its influence on our life force, the most crucial organ of the body: *our heart*. Page after page, one message will rise above all others: our emotions, feelings and breathing patterns determine our destiny. Our very lives depend on them.

Introduction

————— 🖋 —————

Conflict between the passion in our hearts and the reasoning in our heads is certainly a common situation all of us have experienced over and over in our lives. During my training in bioenergetic analysis, I was struck by a dream Dr. Alexander Lowen shared with us. I have asked him to share it again as the opening metaphor for *Heartbreak and Heart Disease*.

—Stephen T. Sinatra, M.D., F.A.C.C

Most individuals in this culture are brought up under the injunction, "Don't lose your head." This means that one must stay in control of one's feelings. Of course, one should be able to control one's actions; but to suppress feeling one has to deaden the body since feeling is the life of the body just as thinking is the life of the head. The most important feeling is love, which is the life beat of the heart. If we are afraid to surrender to love, we imprison our hearts in rigid cages so that they are protected but not free. Without freedom there is no true love and our hearts will languish, as happens to many individuals who are afraid to open their hearts for fear of being hurt.

Too many people have experienced heartbreak in childhood when the love of their parents was tentative and conditional. They no longer trust their hearts or feeling of love. This is the true vulnerability that predisposes them to further heartbreaking experiences of loss of love and eventually to heart disease and death.

About 20 years ago I had a dream that made me aware of my vulnerability. In the dream I was the trusted advisor of an infantile king who believed that I had betrayed him. For this betrayal he ordered that I be executed by having my head cut off. In the dream I saw myself standing next to the execution block beside the executioner with his axe. I wasn't afraid because I believed that the king would realize he was mistaken and that I would receive a last minute reprieve. I could sense the seconds ticking away in the last minute with no reprieve coming. I looked down at my ankles and saw that the chains binding me were tinsel. At that moment I awoke.

It did not take me long to interpret the dream. I sensed immediately that the infantile king was my heart and that I had, in truth, betrayed my heart by listening to the reasoning of my head against the feeling of my heart. The heart may be infantile or childlike in its trust of feeling over reason, but the feelings of the body have guided human action successfully for several million years; reason is a late development in evolutionary history. As Voltaire remarked, "The heart has its reasons which reason cannot comprehend." My faith in the body and its feelings has sustained me over many years. I will never betray my heart.

—Alexander Lowen, M.D.
Author of *Love, Sex and Your Heart*

CHAPTER 1

───── ✍ ─────

My Journey

The Transformation of a Cardiologist/Psychotherapist

It was 3 A.M. in the year 1973. I had just received yet another call during a typically exhausting night during my internship. As I approached the nursing station at Albany Medical Center, many worrisome thoughts went through my mind. Did I have to pronounce somebody dead? Was I going to see a patient dying of cancer? Or perhaps, I simply had to insert a nasogastric tube, start an IV or calm down an anxious patient. It was a year that I will never forget. It was then the days of the "iron men."

This time, I was summoned to see a fragile, elderly man. Unfortunately for us both, he could not speak. His larynx had been removed 24 hours before due to a rapidly growing cancer. Although I was groggy from lack of sleep, I still remember the details so clearly. I was called to start an intravenous line so that this man could continue to receive his medication. What I did not know as I walked into his room was that this man was dying. Even as he was leaving this life, he was reaching out to me. As I took his hand to insert a needle, I saw four letters tattooed above each knuckle. There was the word **L-O-V-E** staring me in the face. As he gave me his hand, he began to communicate in a nonverbal, even spiritual way. As I tried to start the intravenous therapy, he desperately tried to tell me that it was neither what he wanted nor needed.

1

At that time I was a young doctor and believed intellectually that to perform my duty for this man, I had only to administer the antibiotic he needed. What I didn't know then was that all this man really wanted was some human contact.

After starting the intravenous line, I spontaneously held this gentle man in my arms as he rested against my chest. I can still remember how I considered going back to my room to catch a few minutes of much needed rest. But the softer part of me chose to be with him. As I held him, I reflected on his tattoo. I managed to put off a couple of nonurgent calls so I could just sit with him. I started to rock him, assuring him that everything would be okay. Only then, with my arms around him, was he peaceful. While I was holding him, I wasn't performing or evaluating. I wasn't doing anything. I was just being there and offering human contact. As I cuddled and rocked him, there was no threat or struggle. There was a letting down. A short while later, the old man died quietly and peacefully in my arms. It was at that moment I knew that I could no longer be an "iron man."

In those days as *iron men*, we worked throughout the day and night, every second to third night. Some of the doctors, one or two years older than myself, called themselves the real *iron men*. They earned this nickname because they were on call every other night, functioning on only one or two hours of sleep. Those were the days "when men were men," when men performed and achieved efficiently but without feeling. They were tough and insensitive to their own feelings of fatigue and exhaustion. They were, indeed, men of steel and I counted myself as one of them. And the women interns considered themselves women of steel.

We would not realize until much later what this disconnection between performance and feeling—the head and the heart—could ultimately cost each one of us.

But this old man was a special gift to me. For a brief time he took me out of my mind and into my body and its feelings.

He gave me the spiritual message that the act of simple contact and connectedness was an expression of love.

As I pronounced him dead and recorded the time in his chart, I felt I was saying goodbye to a messenger with whom I had a very special encounter. As I left his room, I walked down the hall and started to cry. Crying was a true, genuine feeling that I often suppressed, first as a child, and later as an athlete, college and medical student. At that moment, through my tears, the "voice of my heart"—my feelings, intuition and instincts, rather than my intellect or thoughts, seemed to represent the real truth. It would be many years later before I realized that this moment would be the most valuable and intimate in my training as a physician. These profound unconscious feelings probably directed me into the specialties of cardiology and later, psychotherapy. Perhaps, I was searching for my own "heart feelings." As frequently happens, many of us enter and select professions, searching for answers to our own unresolved, unconscious issues.

As a clinical cardiologist, I have worked with many cases of heart disease. But despite all the studies linking smoking, high levels of blood cholesterol, hypertension and adult diabetes to coronary atherosclerosis, I am convinced that these risk factors, although highly significant, do not fully explain the nature of this illness. Although these risk factors are significant variables in the relationship between lifestyle and cardiovascular disease, additional research studies have confirmed the dominant role of psychological, emotional and metabolic stress in the etiology of heart disease. Appreciating this relationship has become a major challenge for me. Is the heart just a pump to push blood around the body or does it represent something more? This investigation has been my life's quest.

After completing my medical training, I soon began my training as a psychoanalyst. It was then that my real growth in cardiac healing began. After 12 years of study in both Gestalt and bioenergetic psychotherapy, it became clear to me that pathology (becoming ill) is really a form of *dis-ease* that emerges from the chaotic imbalance of mind, body and spirit. Heart disease is the most frequent illness in the Western world resulting from this disturbed relationship.

When considering any illness, diagnosis or treatment, I started to focus not only on the disease and the physical dysfunction created, but also on the human operational planes; the physical, the metabolic, the emotional, the mental and even the spiritual. I soon developed a new appreciation for conscious as well as unconscious drives. The more I learned, the more I realized that to truly be able to help my patients, I needed to be more in touch with energy systems.

The Human Energy System

The healthy operation of the body and its human energy system involves both generative and maintenance phases. Adequate generation depends on the intake of sufficient oxygen and essential nutrients. Maintenance of balance is based on a more complex mixture of environmental variables. A deficiency or an imbalance in any part of the system may contribute over time to the impaired functioning of our cells, tissues, organs and eventually, our bodies. Thus, the concept of energy is both quantitative and qualitative, combining the physical, mental and spiritual realms.

The realization of this combined relationship in healing ignited my interest in exploring these processes thereby integrating optimum health in the whole person. Again, it was my previous training in psychotherapy, emphasizing energetic blocks that opened my eyes to the concept of energy at both the systemic (body) and cellular levels. For example, on the body level, many of us have noticed aggressive, coronary-prone individuals suck in breath during speech even while continuing to speak, exhaling brief sighs and/or muffled grunts when breathing out. Such a disturbance of respiration results in a charged, nonpulsating energetic cycle that consists of fixation on inhalation and constrained mobilization during exhalation which creates difficulties in relaxation during the breathing cycle. Such disturbances in respiratory motility result from chronic body armoring of the chest wall. Tension can be seen in the other body segments as well, including the pelvis, throat and diaphragm. The trapping of energy within the body leads to the inability to breathe freely, experience feelings and release tension. We shall see that such chronic stagnation of energy may render individuals susceptible to heart disease.

Now at the cellular level, similar disturbances of motility occur. When a cell is in a well-nourished, oxygenated, environmentally balanced state, an effortless pulsation occurs. Such a cell is in equilibrium (homeostasis). It is nourished, healthy and perhaps even "happy." But, when a cell becomes contracted due to metabolic, environmental or emotional factors, pulsation is disrupted and healthy functioning is disturbed.

To put this in experimental terms, one can take protoplasm (living matter), place it under a microscope and watch it move. Protoplasm has an energetic pulsating quality; that is, it has a characteristic ebb and flow of its own intrinsic energy. For example, protoplasm may move toward light and warmth, or move away from dark and cold. If a noxious stimulant such as caffeine, aspirin or sulfur dioxide is placed near the medium, what happens? The protoplasm shrinks. It contracts as if trying to protect itself. On the other hand, if a soothing chemical like acetylcholine (a transmitter of the parasympathetic nervous system) is added, the protoplasm expands and moves toward that direction. Aloe vera, a soothing nutrient to the gastrointestinal tract, would probably have the same effect.

This is an important concept in understanding the nature of disease. Our bodies are protoplasm. In simple terms, we expand or contract when encountering environmental forces.

For example, when we are under stress or presented with a noxious stimulus, whether it be a loud noise, extreme cold or rage, we tend to "shut down" and contract all expression of feeling. Similarly, when a child is confronted with negativity from an overpowering parent, the child contracts, shuts off breathing and drives energy within. Even as adults, we may freeze unconsciously in situations of fear, uncertainty or emotional confrontation. It may be compared to a rattlesnake approaching a rabbit. The rabbit, full of fear, freezes and cannot move. Breathing becomes shallow and contracted. Instead of hopping, running and fleeing, the rabbit's fear interrupts the natural ebb and flow of pulsation. Not being integrated, the creature may die holding on to the rigid position. Metaphorically, we shall see in a subsequent analysis that this is a key insight into understanding the nature of coronary heart disease.

Even prehistoric man knew that all life depended upon a pulsating heart. Pulsation is the key element in health. But when pulsation is disturbed or when cells are continuously contracted, energy is drained and constrained, thus enhancing the cells' vulnerability. It is these simple polarities between expansion and contraction that set the stage for the energetic principles of disease.

The health of the body begins to deteriorate when its physical, emotional and mental processes become disintegrated and fail to work in harmony. To establish health and balance within a person, his or her fragmented parts must be reintegrated. This requires a multidisciplinary approach. Such an approach may include elements of proper breathing, exercise, release of painful emotions and past trauma, energy enhancement, nutritional healing, reopening of the heart to love and the development of a spiritual connection.

Investigating all these concepts has been the focus of my personal journey. During my early training in mind/body interactions, I was indeed fortunate to discover many gifted teachers. Seventy years ago Dr. Francis Peabody wrote:

Disease in man is never exactly the same as disease in an experimental animal, for in man the disease at once affects and is affected by what we call the emotional life. Thus, the physician who attempts to take care of a patient while he neglects this factor is as unscientific as the investigator who neglects to control all the conditions that may affect his experiment. The good physician knows his patients through and through, and his knowledge is sought dearly. Time, sympathy and understanding must be lavishly dispensed, but the reward is to be found in that personal bond which forms the greatest satisfaction of the practice of medicine. One of the essential qualities of the clinician is interest in humanity, for the secret of the care of the patient is in caring for the patient.

Caring for the patient is the hallmark of a good physician. But as Peabody suggests, caring incorporates many levels including the physical, emotional and spiritual. It was during my internship in medicine and psychiatry at Albany Medical Center in 1972 that I realized for the first time the ultimate impact of spiritual healing. Although occasional "messengers" were sent to me like my tattooed friend, I soon forgot the deep meaning of these spiritual encounters. Many years later I returned to this vital area. However, during the 1970s I focused primarily on the physical realm of medicine. After my medical residency and cardiology fellowship, I received my board certification in cardiology and entered a very busy practice in clinical cardiology. The next four years of my life I worked long hours in medicine and cardiac diseases. As a highly-trained, technical invasive cardiologist, I felt extremely confident in what I was doing. I became a workaholic. However, the stress of working with acute heart attacks, death and dying, and endless life-threatening emergencies became overwhelming.

Cardiologists—and I was no exception—are particularly vulnerable to heart disease themselves, and not only because of the stressful nature of their work. The personality characteristics of individuals drawn to this highly competitive, high-risk, high-vigilance specialty are those of the coronary-prone individual.

In addition to making second-to-second lifesaving decisions, we frequently have to recommend invasive procedures to our patients which carry the potential for bodily harm. Our vigilance in these situations is sometimes overwhelming. We have to bury feelings and perform like fine-tuned athletes with razor-sharp accuracy and precision. And there is absolutely no room for error.

Back to My Childhood

As a cardiologist, I soon became aware of the patterns of destructive behavior that lay underneath those patients labeled "prone to developing coronary heart disease." For example, I saw many young men with heart disease with driven personalities and passions. But, what I did not expect to discover was that I was wearing this label myself. This awareness was terrifying. I knew that I was competitive, an overachiever and a hard worker, a typical Type-A individual. Thinking was more important to me than feeling.

As a man in my early 30s, aggressive and successful, the reality of my own mortality was suddenly revealed to me through my patients. This realization that I was setting myself up for coronary illness propelled me to investigate transcendental meditation, yoga and even psychotherapy, with a goal to attenuate and soften some of the risky aspects of my behavior. During this time, I recalled what Scott Peck, author of *People of the Lie* and *The Road Less Traveled*, had written about psychotherapy. Peck saw nothing negative about entering therapy. He called this the "high road" of obtaining personal and mental knowledge as well as spiritual growth.

At approximately the same time, Ken Pelletier wrote about the necessity of knowing one's self as a way of impacting others. He stated, "Anyone in a healing profession must become acquainted with his own emotional nature, his personality conflicts, his strengths and weaknesses, and generally to engage in a process of self-exploration." I resonated with these revelations and for the first time developed a hunger for investigating both my conscious and unconscious self.

My search sent me back to my childhood, and a recognizable pattern emerged. I was the third of four children. When I was four years old my sister was born and around that time I succumbed to a series of childhood illnesses and accidents. Were those incidents a maladaptive way to achieve contact and love from a mother who must have had her hands full with a new baby and a growing family?

Through the years I can still feel that yearning for my mother's attention and soothing. Her seeming "unavailability" to me constituted my first heartbreak. The traumatic sadness that followed was repressed but, incredibly, my body remembered the truth. The soft vulnerability of my "child within" evolved into the rigidity of a heavily armored chest, as if to protect my heart. I knew my mother loved me dearly, but at that young age, I was unable to understand her needs and focused only on my own. I sought her approval and love, hoping that by being a "good boy," a good student, an athlete and an achiever, I would win her over. Success would bring me love, I thought. I developed a false connection between the two that carried through to adulthood. This connection lay behind my excessive drive and Type-A behavior that could ultimately cause my premature death.

As a highly trained invasive cardiologist, I felt extremely confident about my ability to perform. My work became my life's passion; provided me with my "place" in the universe. However, over a short period of time, in the midst of this success, I felt myself burning out. I had become locked in an internal struggle to achieve and perform even at the expense of my feelings. Although I didn't recognize it at the time, I had become a driven man. I denied my fatigue, pain and feelings as I had done in my adolescence to prove myself a good student and athlete. In this pursuit of success and achievement, was I really seeking approval and love? Was I trying to prove myself worthy of love? I had carried this need through the years and had seen it manifested again and again in many of my patients. Too many of them had chased this need to heart disease and ultimately to death.

The challenge now before me was the alteration of my own self-destructive, coronary-prone behavior pattern. Actually, the awareness and recognition that I possessed this behavior was enlightening, for it was this awareness that gave me the strength to find a curative alternative.

In the mid 1970's, I attended many lectures and seminars given by my colleagues on behavior and cardiovascular disease. One colleague in particular had a big impact on me— Dr. Robert Eliot, author of *Is It Worth Dying For?* As a cardiologist who had himself suffered a heart attack, Dr. Eliot was intimately aware of the connection between behavior and heart disease. After hearing these lectures, I began attending many self-awareness seminars.

In 1978, I attended an international symposium in London, England on stress and tension. It was extremely provocative and opened me to some of the nontraditional approaches toward healing. While the Americans were teaching stress management in the form of progressive relaxation, the West Germans were integrating biofeedback with their treatments, the Swedes were utilizing massage, the Swiss introduced Lamaze and the Asians focused on meditation. I was able to see each of these methods as a positive way of healing emotion and calming the nervous system. They all had merit, but a piece was missing. Many of these techniques were like taking aspirin for a headache while never exploring the medical source of the pain. My search continued.

The Group Process

Over the next few years, I was asked to help lead stress and illness workshops with internist Dr. Brendan Montano and psychotherapist Holly Hatch. In these group sessions, Holly utilized the Gestalt technique, incorporating Montano's knowledge of the body/mind connection relating to general disease. I contributed my experience of this connection specifically relating to the heart. These group sessions were helpful in teaching susceptible individuals how to cope with life. Group awareness training had a tremendous impact on healing, particularly when individuals saw themselves in other people.

Group process works something like this: Whenever you overreact to other people in group situations, it is because it has triggered an unfinished piece of business in your own psyche. Or, to take this to another level, whatever you don't like in a group member could be something that you don't like in yourself. We all periodically have negative feelings toward others which are actually reactions to hidden aspects of our own characters.

These workshops typically included approximately 18 to 25 people from all walks of life. After a two-hour introductory session concerning the philosophy of stress and illness, a question-and-answer period followed. The focus of these group sessions was the opportunity for participants to look at their own reasons for creating and experiencing stress and tension in their lives. Each person was given the opportunity to examine his or her attitudes and beliefs, with the assistance and feedback of the group leaders. Beliefs and attitudes were also examined through relaxation techniques. These processes led to a further understanding of how each person participates in creating his or her own stress. The response to this awareness ranged from a sense of relief for some to a high level of resistance and anxiety for others. The expression of all emotions was encouraged throughout the seminar, especially during the powerful regression process. This mental process explores stressful experiences during one's early growth and development, particularly during the Oedipal period of one's life, usually four to six years of age. This process resulted in the strongest emotional releases and feelings for many participants.

However, when I attempted this activity, I fell asleep. This happened at least four or five times. Questioning why I fell asleep caused me to dig deeper into my psychological process. Was there something in my early childhood development at approximately five years of age that I didn't want to remember? Later, through years of analysis with Dr. Alexander, Lowen and others, I discovered that my painful experience of heartbreak was something that I really didn't wish to remember. As I buried it in my unconscious, my mind forgot but my body still remembered. In therapy I worked on softening my chest, exploring feeling and enhancing my breathing. Such uncovering of my own heartbreak allowed me to make tremendous strides in connecting with my true self. After my discovery about my own heartbreak, I was able to use my experience to get others in touch with theirs.

I subsequently designed and directed *Healing the Heart* trainings for my patients, where the goal is increasing one's awareness and consciousness through making deeper contact with oneself and others. These workshops last approximately four to five days, using a multidisciplinary approach which incorporates nutritional, psychological and emotional healings. In addition to group process, both Gestalt and bioenergetic psychotherapy, guided mental imagery and other types of meditative processes help to connect the participant to inner heart feelings and emotions.

Gestalt therapeutic techniques that focus on conscious feelings have the potential to bring the individual back in contact with many of his or her bodily emotions. Gestalt also focuses intensely on the present, in the "here and now" experience. There is particular emphasis on breathing and how the interruption of the normal respiratory cycle through fear and other internalized emotions can negatively impact our hearts. After leading several of these sessions, I began to publish some of my own findings on the relationship of stress and disease with particular application to the heart in medical journals.

Two years into my practice as a cardiologist, I decided to

pursue specialized training in the field of psychotherapy. I was amazed at how frequently buried childhood emotions were later expressed in the adult in the form of heart disease. I wanted to learn all I could. The more I read, the more I wanted to know. The connection between mind, emotion and heart was absolutely clear to me. But I still needed to put it all together. The missing piece was the study of personality development, beginning with my own.

For two year I studied Gestalt therapy, including a superficial analysis of myself, which helped me to understand some of the background causes of my attitudes. This investigation further convinced me that the power of emotions is directly related to health and illness. The study of mind and body was so vast and intricate that the more I pursued these relationships, the more uneasy and inadequate I felt. The subject was vast and unexplored.

Although my initial research explored the relationship between stress and illness, my specific interest was the relationship between personality and heart disease and there was little data available on this subject. Actually, throughout my many years of practice, I found that my best teachers were my patients.

Still, I wanted to know if there was something beyond Type-A behavior. Was Type-A behavior just an expression of one's personality? Or, was there something more profound, and worthy of further analysis? Might this be the missing link?

Not only did behavioral analysis become the focus of my interest and energies, it became a challenge. I had begun my search to look for the causative factors that may render one vulnerable to heart disease. The identification and modification of these character traits in order to enhance and prolong life became my purpose. Is the heart merely a pump that pushes blood around the body? Or is it, as the poets say, the home for emotions, passions and feelings? Finding the answers has entailed a quest of over 20 years of medicine and 15 years of bioenergetic analysis. This is why, as a traditionally trained cardiologist, I decided to become a psychotherapist as well. To my knowledge, I am the only certified cardiologist and bioenergetic psychotherapist in the world.

The psychoanalytically based bioenergetic therapy originates from the works of Wilhelm Reich. Reich, an Austrian psychiatrist and a student of Freud, proposed that love, and with it, a healthy sexuality, could cure the ills of mankind. Reich was known for his writings on the relationship of disease, emotions and the denial or absence of pleasure. For example, in *Character Analysis*, Reich described cancer as a resignation from life. He believed that cancer originates in the unreleased feelings of sadness and anger that cause depression.

Recently, it has been verified that emotions do in fact play a major role in cancer. Dr. Bernie Siegel discusses the cancer personality as one who is stuck and willing to give up. Siegel says that "fighting back" through releasing anger and expressing feelings, forgiving and loving the self as well as visualizing the self overcoming the enemy cancer within, is the way to heal. To me, this is very similar to Reich's theory of releasing blocked energy through breathing, kicking, screaming and allowing the body to take over.

Alexander Lowen has spent a lifetime expanding on Reich's theory while developing his own. As a student of Reich, Lowen created the therapy called bioenergetics, a body-oriented analytic therapy focusing on the muscular tensions in the body that are the physical counterparts of the emotional conflict in the personality. Just as one can tell the age of a tree by counting the internal rings on the stump, a bioenergetic therapist, like Lowen, can determine the history of a person by looking at the body. In bioenergetic analysis, the therapist can determine where tension is located and where energy is blocked. The blockage keeps people from experiencing their full potential of aliveness. By utilizing various techniques and exercises to charge and discharge the body, the bioenergetic therapist can release trapped energy, which allows for the dissipation of tension.

Lowen's theory, which incorporates emotional conflict and physical expression in the disease model, appealed to me. As a clinical cardiologist, I was particularly struck by Lowen's focus on breathing in his approach to body therapy. It became more apparent to me that energy and breathing were related to heart disease. Having studied medicine and psychiatry, I decided to study with Lowen and learn some of his techniques, which I now apply to healing the heart. After working with him for two years, he became convinced of this as well and wrote the book, *Love, Sex and Your Heart,* for which I wrote the introduction.

Through Lowen's teachings, it soon became apparent to me that my body was quite tense, that I was not breathing deeply, and that I was not fully experiencing or expressing my feelings. My therapy with Dr. Lowen focused on the rigidity of my body. After the first few years of therapy, my chest and pelvis still remained rigid, armored and under control of my head. Lowen worked on my breathing which induced feeling. The therapy, at times, was painful. He placed me in various positions where my chest would open up and my breathing would be stimulated. He asked me to use my voice in these maneuvers to dissipate the energy in my chest. These maneuvers all had a positive effect in reducing the stress and tension in my chest wall. He then began to focus on my diaphragm, jaw and pelvis.

As months passed by, Lowen persisted but I resisted as if I were a child saying "no" to my father. It was only years later that I realized that softness was the only way to get to the heart of the matter, which in my case was heartbreak. Although strong body techniques used by Lowen have their place, a combination of reaching, softness and tenderness induce vulnerability and tears which finally release long suppressed heartbreak. Crying is nature's way of natural healing. This is the essence of healing the heart. Recently, research has revealed that the crying of emotional tears initiate the hormones that positively stimulate the immune system.

Body-oriented therapy, in my opinion, facilitates the release of old memories stored in the body that continuously solidify the character. I believe that thorough understanding of this concept is the missing link between character and heart disease where the memories are stored in the body as armoring, rigidity and energy blocks. This is the foundation of bioenergetic therapy. According to Lowen, bioenergetic analysis goes beyond releasing these blocked memories to fully experiencing deeper respirations or the breath of life.

Several months of Lowen's body work uncovered my suppressed emotion and released my muscular tension. Gradually, a softening in my body occurred. Crying released tension, inducing an expansive quality in my chest. Over the years, I have found my heart opening. For the first time, I felt I was healing my heart. The growth has been tremendous. The pain of therapy eventually led to the discovery of pleasure. I began to experience more feeling. My emotional and physical well-being heightened and my body seemed to come alive. I began to experience my authentic self. This ongoing journey of self-discovery has been exhilarating.

With these new insights, I began to look at my cardiac patients from a new point of view. I started to observe their chests, the tension located in their bodies and how well they breathed. I inquired into their early life experiences with relation to loss of love, as well as their current experiences with love and intimacy. My work began to evolve to a new, exciting level. I utilized the knowledge I had gained from Lowen to work with patients who were willing to investigate the mind/body connection that I had just discovered for myself.

Bioenergetic analysis became an invaluable tool in the total assessment of each person I encountered in my practice. Although I continued to take a history from a patient, I now began to focus on their breathing, eye contact, the quality of the patient's energy, the feeling in their handshake, the movement of their diaphragm, their tone of voice and signs of held-in emotion in their body. Analysis of the jaw structure, for instance, gave me clues to the level of the patient's held-in anger. Thus, by looking at body structures, I became more aware of patients' issues and illnesses. Focusing on the mind/body interactions, I became a more effective physician and healer.

As my own therapy with Lowen was coming to a close, he convinced me to become a bioenergetic analyst, and recommended a bioenergetic training program. In 1982 I entered the program in Cambridge, Massachusetts. For certification in bioenergetic analysis, a vigorous training program was required. In addition to a five-year training program consisting of eight weekends a year, 200 hours of personal therapy and 60 hours of supervision were required.

The educational program focused on the physical body, character structure, energetic blocks, transference, counter-transference, expression of feeling and investigation of the boundaries of sexuality. It was a time that I still cherish for it was a time that I devoted to the discovery of my authentic self. In my previous training as a physician, I performed like a robot, taking care of others. Now I was nurturing myself. In addition to a very large reading list, similar to any graduate program, the certification process required publishing a paper, attending conferences at the international level and performing therapy under group supervision.

In the Netherlands in 1986, I was fortunate to meet David Bordella, a unique combination of embryologist and bioenergetic therapist. In Boadella's workshop, I was fascinated by his theories of working with the arms as a way of embryologically working with the heart. Boadella told us that the heart was formed during the eighth week of gestation. The lungs were an extension of the mesoderm and endoderm of the heart. Since the arms arose from an extension of the lung, the arms contained the same germ layers that originally came from the heart. Thus, in the adult, simple arm motions are an indirect way of working with the energy of the heart. I realized for the first time *why* some of my patients with heart attacks have arm pain.

Metaphorically, reaching out with your hand and touching someone is also a way of touching someone with your heart. I was so impressed with Boadella's work that I participated in one of his workshops in Switzerland the next year.

During my bioenergetic training, I read many of the works of Alice Miller concerning narcissistic injury in the developing child; this occurs when a parent wants a child to act in a specific way in order to fill a parental need. In other words, *"You do it my way."* As a cardiologist, I saw the ultimate outcome of narcissistic injury as acute heartbreak. I had the exciting opportunity at a Boston Conference to occupy a front-row seat listening to Alice Miller as she answered questions about the theory of childhood developmental issues resulting from unintentional narcissistic parental expectations. I could hardly contain my enthusiasm as I suggested to her that narcissistic injury is ultimately internalized in the child as *"heartbreak."* I felt a strong connection with her as she validated my insight.

After my initial work with Lowen, several years of my personal journey included working on such issues as heartbreak, rigidity and love and intimacy. Dr. John and Joyce Bellis, Dr. Phil Helfaer and Dr. John Pierrakos were my therapists for several years and helped guide me through my journey of unraveling these mysteries of the unconscious. While working through these issues, I realized that I was on a mission of health and healing.

Pierrakos, another student of Reich, reemphazied that disease can be seen in terms of energetic blocks. After doing individual therapy with Pierrakos for over a year, I was able to experience my "dark side." Getting in touch with one's "shadow" is a necessary, yet very difficult, aspect of psychotherapy. I will expand on this later in this text. My therapy with Pierrakos ended in the late 1980's, with the sudden unexpected and heartbreaking death of my father.

On New Year's Eve, 1988, I was supposed to be on a plane to Hawaii. However, my conference was canceled at the last minute and I chose to spend New Year's Eve with my parents. My drive to New York that afternoon was swift and easy. The traffic that I anticipated did not materialize. My expected three-and-one-half hour trip took only two-and-one-half hours. As I approached the driveway of my house, I reexperienced my boyhood feelings of joy at coming home. But as I walked in the door, I heard my father urgently calling my name from upstairs. I ran up the stairs sensing that he was in distress. He was experiencing some pain in his leg and was feeling dizzy. As I came through the door, I could see the look of fear and apprehension on his face, he was sweating. He told me he felt cold and that his leg was "dead." I could feel no pulse there.

I immediately recognized the situation as serious and telephoned his physician. As I walked back to his room, however, he had stopped breathing. I performed CPR furiously; yet I knew that I had lost my father. The shock of the sudden cardiac death left me numb. After all, I had resuscitated many individuals in the emergency room, in the coronary care units and even in hospital wards, bringing many of them back to life. Regardless of how well I had performed the cardiac resuscitation on others, I had failed to save my own father.

I now had the ordeal of telling my mother and calling my siblings. This was even more difficult than the wake and funeral. Since the day after New Year's was a holiday that year, his burial was delayed one day. It was at this time that I felt a tremendous tranquility in my body. I felt as if a spirit had returned to me that I had long since forgotten from my earlier days as a young Catholic boy. At the time of his funeral, I remember hearing the young priest talk about the sudden death of his best friend. His friend had died of a ruptured aortic aneurysm, almost the exact cause of death in my father. At the funeral. I played the Harry Chapin song "*The Cat's in the Cradle*," whose lyrics beautifully capture man's deep yearning to connect with his father. I, as well as other men, wept. Our tears were a way of self-healing. I will never forget the calmness and tranquility I felt. How could I feel such inner calmness in the face of such a drastic and unexpected loss?

The answer is perhaps twofold. First, I made a new vital connection with my own spirituality. Was it a coincidence that my conference was canceled and that the lack of traffic on New Year's Eve in New York enabled me to arrive just as my father was dying, giving me the opportunity to spend the last precious moments of his life with him? Just as a cardiologist frequently has to shock a person's chest with electrical current to restore the heart's normal pulsatile rhythm, the sudden loss of my father shocked me into reality. I returned to my roots. For the first time in years, I reconnected with my faith. Unfortunately, over the years, my time had been consumed with medicine, philosophy and psychotherapy. New-age thinking had led me away from my Judeo-Christian beliefs. Once again, I experienced an opportunity in crisis. I chose to turn the loss of the vital connection to my father into a new openness and awareness and a reconnection with spirituality. Thus, in reestablishing an old connection, I was able to work through my deepest despair and feelings of loss with new opportunity and hope. I felt fortunate indeed.

Secondly, the sudden loss of my father also helped heal my body. That is, the intense crying about my inability to save him facilitated the movement of energy in my chest. The deep sobbing was, in fact, healing. Again I knew I was healing my heart over the loss of my father. Although the rigidity in my chest wall had been lessened through therapy with Lowen, Helfaer and Pierrakos, it took a real-life process of grief to fully open me up into further softening.

After the death of my father, my therapy continued. I decided to enter a rolfing program. Rolfing is an intense body therapy aimed at loosening up the deep tissue spasticities by direct myofacial massage. Rolfing, deep tissue work and massage are all excellent therapies designed to get you in touch with your body and its feelings. I still continue to have monthly rolfing sessions. In addition to loosening up the spasticities in my lower back and pelvis, rolfing also soothes the sympathetic nervous system. Like meditation, yoga, tai-chi, and qi-gong, these alternative therapies have considerable merit in healing the body. They all help to release the deleterious aspects of our tension-filled lives.

Conventional medical care relies on acute crisis intervention, pharmacology and surgery when treating disease. For example, the cardiologist treats an acute heart attack with a multitude of drugs and invasive interventions. In an emergency, such traditional therapy is not only mandatory but also lifesaving for the patient. With life-threatening illness, you want the most highly-trained and experienced cardiologist at your bedside. In fact, for any acute catastrophic illness, every individual would want the most qualified clinician. The educational training of a physician in this country requires an incredible commitment of time and energy, a minimum of seven years of postgraduate study. For me, it was actually nine years of postgraduate training. For other more specialized M.D.'s such as cardiovascular surgeons, neurosurgeons and angioplasty cardiologists, it may require as much as 11 years. There is no other profession I know of that requires this much study, education and commitment. Even lawyers, accountants, engineers and rocket scientists do not have the intense physical and emotional training that a physician has in this country.

For this reason, I have a deep respect for any physician who has undergone this process. However, not all of the world's physicians are trained in this manner.

A few years ago a cardiologist from the Soviet Union came to observe my practice. Unfortunately, she had to leave her country due to religious persecution. As a "trained cardiologist," she came to work with me for a time to improve her English and eventually open up her own practice. After the first day, it became quite clear to me that, although this Russian physician knew some aspects of cardiology, she had very little background in clinical cardiology. I inquired about her training. She told me that she underwent six years of combined college and medical school, followed by a one-year internship. Then she took her exams. Since she scored highest in cardiology, she became the attending cardiologist at Hospital #6 in one of the provinces of the Soviet Union.

I was shocked and dismayed that she had had such minimal clinical training and that the speciality of cardiology had been chosen for her. In this country, physicians are required to complete at least three years of internal medicine followed by a minimum of three years of specialized training in cardiology to receive board eligibility in cardiology. This is quite a contrast to the training of a cardiologist in the Soviet Union. The training of a specialized American physician is time-consuming, vigorous and in most cases, very complete. Traditional training, indeed, has outstanding merit and is absolutely required as a base from which to work. However, traditional training, even in America, does have some major weaknesses.

In fact, a recent article in *The New England Journal of Medicine* showed that one out of every three Americans chose unconventional, alternative therapies for their illnesses, spending an additional 14 billion dollars annually. Although many were using nutritional remedies, such as vitamins, minerals and herbs, a third of these individuals surveyed were seeing alternative caregivers. It is interesting to note that in this particular group, approximately 80 percent of these individuals were also seeing an orthodox physician for the same illness. However, most of them (72 percent) had not told their doctors about the alternative care practitioner. The bottom line is that Americans made more visits to alternative caregivers in 1990 than they had to all types of primary care physicians. Many of these therapies consisted of lifestyle changes including alterations in diet, use of supplements, managing stress and focusing on techniques to enhance breathing such as yoga and relaxation therapies. Other mind/body approaches included visualization, prayer and music therapies.

I have encountered many patients who simply want to improve the quality of their lives via these techniques. For example, consider my patient Mary.

Mary believed that she had the power within herself to help heal her heart. Unfortunately, when she addressed this issue with her cardiologist, she was told that there was nothing that she could do to help herself other than continue with her present medical therapies and, if her disease worsened, she could consider a possible heart transplant. Mary desperately wanted to have an active role in her healthcare. Feeling frustrated by the answers she was getting from her physician, an excellent conventional cardiologist, she decided to see me.

When I first saw Mary, she told me that she wanted a traditional cardiologist who could "complement" her care. After we spoke and I examined her, I felt that there were certainly some natural healing therapies that could be of benefit to her. I suggested nutritional supplements including coenzyme Q^{10}, magnesium and my antioxidant vitamin/mineral formula in addition to her current medications. I also suggested that Mary change her diet and incorporate mental imagery into her daily routine. This way, she could actually visualize her heart healing. These suggestions not only helped Mary physically, but emotionally and spiritually as well. Perhaps the most important aspect of Mary's healing was that she had hope, which was critical for healing herself. With a combination of conventional and complementary therapies, Mary had a significant improvement in the quality of her life.

The problem with standard allopathic care in our country is that it is crisis-oriented, or in simpler terms, a Band-Aid fix. Consider the use of aspirin for a headache. Although aspirin offers some relief of pain, it doesn't address the underlying cause of the headache nor does it help the patient to prevent future headache. The typical model of medicine in this country is based on trying to fix and administer relief with pharmacological, surgical and other interventions.

In heart disease, the real healing needs to take place *after* the bypass or angioplasty has occurred. Although these treatments may buy time for the patient to heal, bypass and angioplasty procedures are not cures. In reality, they are only "aspirin for a headache." Like Mary and millions of Americans like her, many patients want something more than standard allopathic care. Over the last few years, I have been seeing more and more patients who want to take responsibility for their own health and participate in their own healing.

Getting well requires that the physician and the patient share in the healing process as a team. We must remember what truly heals—*nature, time* and *patience*. Paracelsus, a physician during the reformation, stated, "*Nature cures, the doctor only nurses.*" Although patients have the power to enhance their healing, it is the role of the physician to help stimulate and nurture that power and mobilize the intrinsic forces in the patient that offer resistance to disease. A good physician is one who will assist patients to find and stimulate their own healing powers.

Healing, therefore, is a commitment between physician and the patient engaging the mind, body and spirit. On the other hand, there are some patients who do not wish to enter equal interactive relationships with their doctors. As Gerald Epstein wrote in his book, *Healing Immortality*, some of the lonely and elderly cling to their old dependencies, finding it essential to rely on contact with their doctor. Sometimes a visit to their doctor is the only contact they have. For many of the elderly, this is the only vital connection in their lives. Although this is tragic and most unfortunate, the alienated and lonely sustain this contact by staying sick. Thus, they become dependent on their physician for survival. As victims, they feel so helpless and depleted they want the doctor to literally "fix them" and do all the work without their participation in their own healing. Many physicians get trapped in this codependent relationship as well. Role reversal occurs with the physicians who, while trying to fill every need of this codependent relationship, now become victims to their own patients. This relationship can deteriorate into an action/reaction modality. Thus, integrated healing fails to occur.

The problem with typical allopathic medicine is that it does not educate physicians to support balanced interactive relationships between themselves and their patients. For example, if the allopathic physician completely takes over, the patient's inner healing ability will be stifled. I have seen many physicians completely take over a patient's care, feeling that their remedies will "cure" the patient. Rigid overcontrol can be the Achilles heal of the modern physician.

Although most of my colleagues have been exposed to complementary therapies, many of them have continued to maintain an arrogant and negative attitude toward them. Unfortunately, this personal bias may block real healing. When a patient is being treated and there is a narcissistic need in a physician to completely take control, the patient's own inner healer will remain unawakened. This is frequently the case in cardiac disease.

Although some cardiologists counsel their patients about

risk-factor modification, many cardiologists really do not have the time or the patience to investigate the profound behavioral aspects of cardiology. In my studies as a psychotherapist, I began to appreciate the deeper processes through which health is maintained, lost, regained and often lost again. This prompted me to direct my energies more toward preventive medicine which consisted of looking deeper into lifestyle, nutritional needs, emotional and psychological factors as well as relationship needs. Over time, I started to acknowledge my own path: *I was an allopathic physician in recovery.*

In addition to treating heart attacks with traditional approaches I am now more interested and committed to exploring all the many reasons why a patient suffers a heart attack in the first place. After physical recovery, I attend to the patient's nutritional, emotional and psychological needs.

We need to ask ourselves the question, Are there certain emotional or psychological constitutional weaknesses in individuals that make them more vulnerable to cardiac events later on in life? Or is heart disease just the result of a maladaptive lifestyle and perhaps an extension of our personalities and characters? We know that one's psychological vulnerability to heart attack and sudden death can arise from a combination of factors including stress, emotional arousal, intense psychological and emotional needs, depression and/or dissatisfaction with life. In addition, coronary heart disease also reflects on the unconscious search for one's true self. Any life-threatening disease or catastrophic illness can cause an incredible shift in one's emotional and psychological nature, bringing one to a new awareness of who he or she really is.

Heart disease has offered many of my patients a new window of opportunity to look deeper into their emotional and spiritual selves; it has allowed them to take what Scott Peck calls *"the road less traveled."* Many of my patients enter psychotherapy as a way of obtaining insight into the reasons behind their cardiac illness. When these issues are uncovered and investigated, these patients discover for themselves not only why they developed heart disease but why they developed it at a particular time. Heart disease often offers an opportunity for a second chance in life. It is a time for patients to finally face and examine lifelong tensions, anxieties, longings and even the hidden, forgotten memories of childhood heartbreak.

Heartbreak is never listed as a cause of disease because it is not considered a medical condition. As a result of a long-term painful experience, from poor parenting to abandonment, a child may partially close his or her heart. Partially closed means that the reaching out to establish another loving connection is hesitant, tentative and never total. When we talk of hearts being closed or open, it sounds "psychological" rather than "physical." But can the psychological ever really be separated from the physical? To make such a separation is to split the unity of the organism as it splits the unity of the healing approach.

A living body is not made up of a psyche and a soma; these are merely two different ways of looking at and talking about the living process. No psychiatrist limits him or herself only to what goes on in the mind of a patient since he or she is aware of the physical processes that largely determine human interactions. By the same token, no cardiologist should confine him or herself only to the physical processes of the heart. To do so is to ignore the fact that the heart is but one part of a total being that functions as a whole. There is no illness that is not physical and mental at the same time, since it is the whole person who is sick. The psychiatrist and the cardiologist can bring their special expertise to the problem of coronary heart disease, but we must recognize that each has a limited approach. Combining the two is what is needed to provide an understanding of cardiac illness in terms of the whole person. Thus, if emotional factors operating on a psychological level affect the disease process, coronary heart disease represents a behavioral disorder. Love, and all its ramifications, represents the nucleus of the problem. Love is also the solution.

Let us consider, on a physical basis, the concept of the heart being open or closed to love. The idea of opening and closing is not alien to the heart whose valves open and close to pump blood throughout the body. Opening and closing also applies to the arteries, the channels through which the blood flows. Healthy arteries, by virtue of the smooth muscle cells in their walls, can open and close to direct blood to areas of special need.

However, when there is disease, plaque forms which partially closes the arteries and limits the flow of blood through them. If there is a significant reduction in blood flow through the coronary arteries, the heart will suffer. The closure of one of these arteries results in a myocardial infarction or heart attack. Atherosclerosis of the coronary arteries is a dominant form of heart disease and a major cause of death.

I deeply believe that there is a connection between childhood heartbreak and coronary heart disease. Heartbreak is defined as a loss of love and intimacy in life. It can result from rejection, whether real, misperceived or even imagined at vulnerable stages of one's life. A closed, guarded heart coupled with the eternal need to take in love, results in a behavioral pattern that over the years eventually puts the heart at risk. Thus, it can be hypothesized that a closed heart or a heart without love is prone to heart disease. It is important to understand this mind/body connection so that we may see how our emotional lives are tied to our physical well-being. The first step is to examine the nature of heartbreak as a coronary risk factor.

CHAPTER 2

Heartbreak: A Coronary Risk Factor

On a day-to-day basis, most of us are casual about the workings of our bodies until there is a breakdown somewhere and we are called to attention by whatever part we have offended, letting us know that we have been caught. Gallstones, ulcers and lost teeth are signs that map our lives and categorize our behavior patterns, displaying our inattention and neglect to our body. Frequently the first recognized symptom of heart disease is sudden death. There is no chastisement, no warning to mend our ways, no trade-off or time to bargain with our fate. This omnipotent organ demonstrates its power over us with one unforgiving defense maneuver. It attacks us.

Coronary artery disease is the most common cause of death in the industrialized world. In its most common form, coronary thrombosis, blood clots in strategic vessels of the heart withhold oxygen to the heart muscle, resulting in injury to the muscular walls of the heart. This may precipitate ventricular fibrillation, a state in which the chamber of the heart that propels blood to the brain and the body beats as fast and wildly as the wings of a wounded bird, allowing little movement of blood through the arteries.

What have we done to so wound ourselves, to cause this wild flight? Where and when does it begin? How can we change the patterns and the causative factors before it is too late? These are the questions which challenge the contemporary cardiologist who seeks to prevent as well as treat these life-threatening conditions. The answers more and more frequently point toward the necessity of identifying and challenging how we act and how we react, not only in stressful situations, but in everyday life situations.

Our world is filled with situations and happenings, some more important than others. Hunger and deprivation are unquestionably more important than a flat tire, except for the individual who has to deal with a flat tire on a deserted road late at night and with no jack. One would think a failing grade would be more important to a college student than a bad haircut unless perhaps the style damages an already low self esteem. In these cases, the flat tire and the bad haircut can be considered external stressors in these persons' lives. How they respond to these and other stressors will determine their body's physiological reaction and ultimate health.

A stressor is something to which special weight and significance has been attached. Stress occurs when there is a resistance of the body and mind to external stressors. It represents an individual's response to threat, demand or change. Stress can be something as simple as the feeling of being overwhelmed—the inability to give in to a situation, a fear of losing control, or it can be a feeling of struggle or uncertainty. Often a stressor cannot be changed or even controlled. What can be controlled, however, is the patient's behavioral response to the external stressor. When the promotion does not come, when the tire goes flat, when the haircut is unattractive, an individual has only two choices—adapting or maladapting. He can adapt by "going with the flow," accepting the situation or working to effect some kind of change. Or he can maladapt by preparing his body for "combat" or for visceral vascular readiness by either withdrawing or by pushing beyond normal expectations in an effort to make the stressor go away. Sometimes maladaptability is exhibited when coping styles are unhealthy and inappropriate such as in drug or alcohol abuse, overeating or overworking. These activities, in themselves, take an enormous toll on the body.

Today's stressed individuals cannot "fight or flee," which was an effective mechanism used by our ancestors. Within the confines of a sophisticated and demanding society, most people accept external stresses by putting their bodies in a chronic state of preparedness. The chronic alarm reaction that develops is a harmful response in which the body continuously overdoses on its own biochemicals.

When the body enters into this modern fight-or-flight response, adrenalin is released, raising the blood pressure, increasing the heart rate, speeding up breathing. If the body remains in this chronic alarm action state for any length of time, it becomes vulnerable to any of a number of physical problems ranging from aching neck muscles and headaches to ulcers, allergies, diminished sexual desire—and cardiovascular disease.

The biochemical alterations that occur in response to stress are powerful, and physicians have long been witness to both the physiological and psychological consequences of stress. When these responses are inappropriate or ineffective, the individual develops "distress." If one cannot find an appropriate adapting mechanism to a particular stressor, he or she, by necessity, must maladapt. Pathological changes can occur in the body because of this maladaption and disruption in hormonal secretions can be long-term and even permanent.

Much of the answer in dealing with stress lies not in the stressors themselves, but in an individual's response to these stressors, i.e., the behavioral response and coping style. An important step in learning how to adapt is to recognize some of the situations that create stress. These can be lack of communication, unfulfilled expectations, retirement, death of a loved one, job pressures, bad relationships and particularly important, dwelling upon past events or imagined future ones. Dwelling on "what might have been" or how life will change with future imaged events may influence stress biochemicals. So often a patient will tell a physician, "my life will work when I retire" or "my life is going to be okay when I get divorced" or "when I change my job, things will begin to change." These projections keep the body in a constant state of anticipation and the eventual reality of unfulfilled expectations has a devastating effect on the body.

A great deal of stress can result when an individual denies responsibility and reacts to a situation by saying "such and such has been done to me." In reality, nobody can make another person feel inadequate, unhappy, unloved or guilty. These feelings and insecurities come from within and are drawn in from outside sources only when they confirm an inner belief. The immediate stress can only be relieved if the person removes himself from the external situation that reflects these attitudes. A healthful response will only come when individuals begin to alter their own attitudes and beliefs about themselves.

An employee says, "my boss always makes me feel inadequate." In truth, the boss does not make the employee feel inadequate; the boss does, however, serve to enhance the employee's already established feelings of inadequacy. The employee reacts by becoming tense and hostile whenever the boss is around. Changing jobs will not alleviate the problem; it will only surface again at the next job. The only way for the employee to change the situation is to develop positive attitudes about himself and his capabilities.

Behavioral research studies have shown that one's personality and how one responds to environmental and/or emotional stresses are extremely important variables in the nature of disease. Sufficient data now exist revealing that chronic exposure to emotional stress and turmoil may lead to biochemical changes in the body which may eventually expose one to pathological conditions. One's personality, character, consciousness and adaptability may determine why one individual responds to a stressful event by developing disease while another does not.

Consider coronary heart disease, a unique phenomenon of contemporary man. According to conventional medical wisdom, atherosclerosis is propagated by a mosaic of physical variables and cardiovascular risk factors, i.e. smoking, high cholesterol, increased blood pressure, to mention a few. But there is more to it than that. The origin of this dreaded disease resides as well in modern man's character and behavior. But we must again ask, why? This behavior is often the result of unresolved emotional conflicts, psychological injuries and developed patterns which unconsciously attack the systems of our bodies.

It might be suggested that today's disease-prone individuals must cope with stressors that were unknown to past generations, such as the highly competitive nature of our society, rapidly changing social mores and environmental imbalances. The threat of war and worldwide destruction is ever present. The 20th century personality is ready to communicate and compete at any given moment. Our business and leisure time is highly structured, active and competitive. Relaxation, casual conversation, and unhurried pleasures are the true luxuries today and are hard to come by. Everyone is in a hurry. Everyone is on the move. The typical modern-day personality exhibits what has come to be known as "Type-A" coronary-prone behavior, whose hallmark qualities are zealous ambition, narcissism, competitiveness and hostility.

Coronary-prone individuals, driven by achievement and performance, strive to succeed without satisfaction or fulfillment. They suppress and deny self-expression. Thinking becomes more important than feeling. They frequently have an overcommitment to work and have a profound sense of time urgency and impatience. Success and a positive self-image are projected to the outside world, while the realities of poor self-esteem, depression and various forms of sexual inadequacy are frequently hidden.

Subconsciously, those at risk for heart attack have a strong desire to control events and many of them experience a need to accomplish out of a profound sense of panic. This internal fury and state of relentlessness are characteristic of the 20th century coronary-prone personality. But, again, it can be asked: Why is there an inordinate drive for success? How did this behavior develop? What function does this serve in personalities? If one does not know what drives one, one cannot act effectively to limit the drive to a reasonable level. If one can understand how these forces act in their personality, specific actions can be taken to diminish their power and so protect the heart from their harmful effects.

In 1974, Meyer Friedman came to the conclusion that the lack of love or unconditional love was responsible for Type-A coronary-prone behavior. Few people would admit that they were unloved as children. Even patients in analysis have considerable difficulty accepting this possibility. Generally it is only after they have experienced the pain of their heartbreak that they are willing to recognize that one or both parents had profound negative feelings towards them. Parental love is a reality of human nature. Unfortunately, it is not the full reality of human life.

Type-A coronary-prone behavior develops in a family situation in which love for the child is conditional upon the child's accomplishments and achievements. In Western cultures, where success has become our most important "virtue," many parents see their child's success as as fulfillment of their own narcissistic desires. Too often, the parents' egos are involved in their children's status and performance in and out of school, in studies and in sports. But love that is conditioned upon performance is not love at all. Conditional love always carries with it the possibility that at some time or another children may experience a withdrawal of parental love if their behavior has not fulfilled parental expectations.

Unconditional love, on the other hand, carries the message that the child is loved for who he or she is and not for what he or she does. If young children receive the message, "You are not acceptable the way you are," basic insecurities develop. These are the basis for the Type-A personality which drive people to achieve as a way to overcome low self-esteem due to their early rejections. If children close their hearts to avoid subsequent rejection and heartbreak, they pay the price of loneliness. Loneliness results in a fear of loving and a fear of new connections. If approval is based on performance or achievement, there is an avoidance of intimacy, contact and commitment. Hoping to gain acceptance and acknowledgement, first at home, then at school and later in the workplace, children falsely assume that successful endeavors will buy them love. In the pursuit to gain lost parental love and overcome such feelings of heartbreak, children sacrifice the true self for an illusion—*success*. Work, performance and this new substituted passion for success displace lost love.

With the ultimate goal of achievement and performance, they strive for success, power and control There is no room for the authentic self in this scenario. Unfortunately, coronary-prone individuals do not see their "striving for success" as an expression of their need for lost love. They do not reach out for love since they are too frightened by the possibility of rejection. They strive to earn love by achievement, performance and success. But this desperate striving is tinged with hidden hostility, aggressiveness and bitterness that prevents others from loving them.

Both Alice Miller and Alexander Lowen argue that some vulnerable place in the child knows the truth. This "true self" has been sacrificed in an attempt to gain approval from the parent. To sacrifice the self is a betrayal of the self. Such a crushing experience results in a narcissistic injury or heartbreak laying the foundation for a character structure and personality that has an acute fear of rejection. With such a tentative fear of reaching toward others, there is a lack of commitment and conviction resulting in an inability to take in love when it occurs. Although the memory of the heartbreak is repressed in the form of denial, the body reveals the truth in its somatic expression. That is, one's chest will be held high and overinflated as if to say, "I don't need your anymore." There is also shallow mechanical breathing, a contraction in the throat and pelvis and a generalized state of body rigidity.

This physical defense against the pain of lost love takes the form of immobilization and rigidification of the chest wall. Unfortunately the defense itself becomes a chronic negative factor in the body over time. It restricts breathing and creates muscular tension, both of which are cardiac stressors. As one's breathing is limited by such chronic tension, one's energy is also limited and less available to deal with other stressors. Research in Eastern Europe has demonstrated this typical pattern of coronary-prone individuals in pulmonary function testing. The pulmonary function tests of these individuals indicate an increased expiratory reserve volume and a decreased inspiratory reserve volume typical of a more inflated chest.

Experimental studies have also demonstrated that as one increases breathing, one increases the hormone prostacycline (PG12) which is an antagonist to the sticky substance of blood platelets or the hormone thromboxane (TX2). Thus, highly mechanical, overinflated breathing not only affects the chest wall in creating a cardiac stress, but also exerts a metabolic stress on the biochemistry of blood clotting. Heartbreak can literally hurt the heart. Heartbreak is directly and indirectly responsible for many cases of heart disease. What could be more direct than the sudden, unexpected death of an individual upon learning of the loss of a loved one?

More common and more subtle, heartbreak is indirectly responsible for heart disease through a body attitude of rigidity and mechanical, chaotic and disturbed breathing patterns. In addition, the pain of longing for a loved one who is not available is heartbreaking. This in itself is a profound stress that affects the core of our being, our heart.

I believe that heartbreak is a profound unconscious issue inherent in every one of us. Heartbreak, loss of love, grief and anguish are certainly a part of life that we all must face at one time or another. Although some of these feelings can be manifested in our consciousness, for most of us they are deeply buried and hidden. Many of these feelings originate during very early stages of growth and development. We have all experienced loss of vital connections and other heartfelt relationships on both the physical and emotional levels. Although some of these losses may be final, as in the death of a loved one, many are not.

In my case, it is quite clear that I experienced heartbreak from ages four-and-a-half to six-and-a-half. My heartbreak began after my sister was born. As a little boy, deeply connected to my mother, I felt that I was "dropped" as her energies were directed to my newborn sister. As a five-year-old, I could not understand the realities and responsibilities of being a parent. I am sure that my mother had her hands full with a newborn and three other young children. But the emotional detachment and perceived "threat of loss" was heartbreaking for me, especially since I was at the height of love and sexuality during the vulnerable Oedipal period of my life. I buried the feelings of heartbreak and tried to buy love by being a good boy and becoming a high achiever. I am sure my choice to become a doctor had its roots in not getting these childhood needs met. I have often said that I probably became a cardiologist as a metaphorical way of looking for my own heart. Fortunately, in psychotherapy, I was able to determine the real reason behind my driven Type-A behavioral pattern.

Heartbreak can be experienced on many levels. For me it

was a simple developmental issue originating during a very vulnerable period in my life. For some, it can be the absolute loss of a vital connection at a very early age both in the physical and emotional sense. Let me tell you about the case of Laszlo.

Laszlo is a 55-year-old male who came into my office for the first time in April, 1995. During one visit, Laszlo asked mè about the portrait of my great-grandfather which hangs in my office. He told me that portrait looked very much like his own father.

As we discussed this further, I noticed that Laszlo began to experience sadness. His voice became lower in tone and his eyes began to water. He told me that he was born in Hungary and had last seen his father when he was three years old. His little boy memories included seeing his father being taken away into Hitler's army. During the war, his father was captured by the Russians and subsequently died of starvation in Siberia two years later. Throughout his childhood and his entire adult life, Laszlo experienced, on an unconscious level, a deep unfulfilled longing for his father. Although he felt some sadness consciously, his unconscious feelings were considerably stronger and more profound. When he developed heart disease in his late 40's and needed triple coronary artery bypass by age 50, he was shocked and dismayed because he had none of the usual risk facotrs associated with heart disease. That is, he was a nonsmoker, had a normal cholesterol level, had no history of hypertension, and there was no known history of coronary artery disease in his family.

But what Laszlo didn't connect with was that a deep longing for an unavailable loved one can, literally, affect the health of the heart. For more than 50 years, Laszlo, on both the conscious and unconscious levels, had painfully longed for his absent, deceased father. He experienced a heavy heart which later manifested as heartbreak. Even though, like many others, he ignored the emotional pain, the physical components of his profound heartbreak were manifested in the body.

As I talked with Laszlo, I noticed that his breathing was shallow, his chest was rigid, and his shoulders were rounded. As we continued to talk I noticed that the energy in his chest was minimal and that he was hardly breathing.

The contours of his chest muscles made it appear that he was wearing a heavily armored chest plate. Laszlo had built up this "armor" as a way to protect his vulnerable childhood heart. As he grew up, his body continued to add to this muscular tension that put a chronic strain on his posture and breathing patterns. His condition is typical of many cardiac patients who have suffered crushing heartbreaks early in their lives. Such emotional feeling, which manifests itself in the body, creates an undue stress on the heart. The rounded shoulders, the rigid chest muscles, and the shallow breathing protected Laszlo from feeling the deep pain and heartbreak of the unremitting longing for his father. But in the end, what had protected the little boy from these painful feelings nearly killed him as an adult.

To avoid the deep anguish of heartbreak, Laszlo unconsciously and chronically deadened the breathing patterns in his body. When breathing is diminished, the capacity for feeling is also diminished. Thus, his heart became "locked" into a frozen chest.

Laszlo's condition arose from unconscious denial patterns that accompanied his profound heartbreak. It is crucial to understand this if we are to understand our own susceptibility to cardiovascular disease.

Consider the issue of denial. Denial is clearly a cardiovascular risk factor. As a cardiologist, I have treated hundreds of patients who were in total denial, not only of their symptoms of heart disease, but even of heart damage itself. Why do patients with heart disease place themselves in situations of such vulnerability? Why do patients push above and beyond their normal expectations? Perhaps it is because denial becomes strong and rooted in their characters from a very early age.

Early rejections on issues of love and sexuality can, indeed, cause heartbreak. Since the loss of love can be so devastating to a child, on some level the child may feel that he/she could actually die. In therapeutic terms, this is called a "death layer" experience. The only way to survive such intense feelings is to forget, block and bury these feelings, thereby denying the emotion of heartbreak in the first place. As I have counseled many patients regarding heart disease, I have come to realize that patients prefer to experience physical pain rather than uncover hidden emotional trauma. However, as we shall see, the investigation of early heartbreak is essential before healing can take place. Although denial on the surface seemingly offers protection, in reality denial of feeling places one in a tremendous state of vulnerability. Since denial is an unconscious mechanism used to control our feelings, it blocks the perception of impulses. Feelings, therefore, become bottled up and many individuals eventually can implode by having a heart attack or explode like a volcano erupting with lava. Thus, many patients who suppress feelings possess the polarity of overreaction to feeling. Anger, for example, which can start as a healthy emotion, may explode into rage, a dangerous and irrational response. I have seen this reaction in many of my patients; one totally dissected his aorta in a fit of rage. We shall investigate this case study in a subsequent chapter.

The vulnerability that stems from denial also weakens our sense of self. When feelings are denied without a solid sense of our emotional self, we become vulnerable if we push beyond our normal expectations. So many of my patients have set the stage for their own heart attacks by picking up a refrigerator, pushing a car or working themselves to death. This denial of self is so characteristic of heart attack patients. It is a suppression of true deep feeling or a denial of reality that contributes to coronary-prone behavior and subsequent cardiovascular risk. This lack of awareness by adults established in childhood is very typical of coronary-prone patients. I believe that core needs unmet in childhood become the unful-filled needs of the adult and that this is the underlying causative factor, the pivotal focus upon which these lives re-volve, dictating behavior and ultimately physiological disease.

Love and Connectedness

Most physicians may not see the connection between heart-break and heart disease because heartbreak is not a recognized condition, just as love is not a recognized physiological func-tion. In the interest of science, physiology has limited itself to mechanics, chemistry and organ function and has ignored the feeling states associated with those functions. Science has been necessarily confined to phenomena that can be objec-tively demonstrated and measured. Feeling states are subjec-tive experiences that lie outside the realm of science, but we cannot exclude them from our understanding of human func-tioning. Love is a tremendously vital force in human behavior and one must try to understand its nature.

Nowhere is the nature of love and connectedness more clearly manifested than in the relationship of a mother and child. A mother's love begins with a physical connection be-tween the embryo and the mother via the umbilical cord. That connection is essential to the life and development of the fetus. At term, the child is born and that physical connection is broken. This break would be fatal to the child if a new con-nection were not made with the mother on a different level. This is best exemplified by the act of nursing. The connection here is between breast and mouth and skin with skin. It is significant that the infant's need for the new connection is announced and communicated by the utterance of a cry, at once demanding and imploring.

As we shall see, crying is necessary if heartbreak is not to lead to heart disease. During infancy the baby will cry every time it experiences a threatened break in its connection to the mother, if it is fearful or has a need it wants met. The growing independence of the child is reflected in its ability to establish connections with persons other than the mother. This is a process that does not stop. Throughout life, we are constantly making new connections on many levels, deeply to some, less deeply to others. In this process, old connections can be strained and some may be broken. But, every break of a connection, whether between friends, parents or lovers, entails pain. Although such necessary losses may allow for more growth and expansion, a break of a vital connection can induce tremendous pain on both physiological and psychological levels.

As adults, most of us establish a deep connection with another person through the sexual act which is appropriately called "making love." When the connection is only sexual, involving the surfaces of two bodies without love or emotional exchange, it is superficial and unfulfilling. The role of the heart, in this case, is merely a mechanical pump, responding only minimally on an emotional level. But the heart is a living pump and is influenced by our feelings, fantasies, passion and connections to other people. These elements create a synergy among physical, mental and emotional responses which we call *love*. "Making love" not only establishes our connections, it reinforces them. The passion of love or the pain of loneliness may affect the heart rate and blood pressure, ultimately affecting the pumping action and the health of the heart.

Many cases on record attest to heartbreak being directly responsible for heart disease. As mentioned earlier, we have all heard of cases of "sudden death" occurring on hearing the news of the death of a loved one. What happens is that such intense feelings affect the heart and heart rhythm. Poetically speaking, the heart and the mind have always been considered interchangeable, but until recently, medical science did not pay much attention to the connection between the two. Now, doctors and researchers are beginning to see a greater connection between the heart and the brain. In a subsequent chapter, we shall see that lethal conversations at times can exist between the brain and the heart. Today, some cardiologists speak not only of angina, arrhythmia or heart attack, but also of heartache: the result of the loss of vital relationships. This heartache can eventually lead to heartbreak, or the literal breaking down of heart function.

Statistics clearly prove that married people have a lower incidence of heart attacks than single or widowed persons. Widowed persons, however, tend to develop disease at an alarming rate, particularly soon after the loss of a loved one. Divorced people are more vulnerable to illness and cardiovascular problems than married people. James Lynch strongly believes that loneliness predisposes an individual to heart trouble. He points out that simple human contact, even simply holding a person's hand has a beneficial effect, making the individual more resistant to the negative effects of threat, danger or uncertainty. Many times in situations of crisis, I have just held a person's hand in an attempt to ameliorate fear and anxiety.

Similar beneficial effects of simple contact have been shown in animal studies. Lynch, for example, has pointed out the estimable value of having pets, particularly dogs. In clinical studies, he showed that the survivors of heart attacks who came home to loyal, nonjudgmental pets had an increased survival rate over those who experienced social isolation and loneliness. Similar data were reported in the *New England Journal of Medicine*, suggesting that loneliness was a major factor in subsequent death of survivors of myocardial infarction. Lynch has also pointed out that living alone is also a coronary risk factor. For example, in 1960 Nevada had the highest risk of heart disease in the U.S. and also the highest rate of divorce.

Lynch also refers to a study of the inhabitants of a Pennsylvania town whose dietary habits included food that was rich in cholesterol and saturated fatty acids, yet the incidence of heart disease in this community was less than the national average. He attributes this finding to the fact that this is a homogenous community of Italian immigrants in which the family relationships have been relatively stable. Such "cultural protection" can also be seen in the cultures of Japan, Yugoslavia and Greece where heart disease is uncommon. If emotional support and love of family are stabilizing to the heart, then by the same token, it can be hypothesized that unstable love relationships can subject an individual to great emotional stress which will in turn negatively impact on the function of the heart.

Here again, it must be pointed out that we are dealing with statistical indications in these studies. Why would being single predispose one individual to cardiac disease but not another? We have all known single people who have lived to a ripe old age. Just as some single persons may have full lives, some married individuals die prematurely due to a fatal heart attack. If it is not a fatal heart attack, it can be an injury that seriously weakens the heart, predisposing it to further attacks which could then be fatal. If loneliness is such a potent emotional stressor that it could lead to heart disease, why doesn't marriage serve as a protection? It can be argued that just as one can be quite lonely in a crowd, so can one feel cut off and isolated in a marriage where there is no real communication between the partners. There are marriages where over the years spouses say little more than formal words to each other. One could understand the feelings of loneliness a husband or wife could have in such a situation. Sometimes the loneliness is alleviated by outside relationships, each spouse going his or her own way. In other marriages, one can sense the hostility between the partners which may be expressed in scornful looks, shouts, or even physical violence. Yet, even the spouses who seem to survive in spite of the continuing stress of bad feelings will eventually experience a breakdown in their health.

Heart disease, for many, begins in the home. As a clinical cardiologist, I have often heard statements like, "I'm married to a stranger" or "I'll stay in this marriage if it kills me." Unfortunately, that was the case for John:

John, a man in his early 40's, came in for consultation because of marked fatigue, depression and difficulty sleeping. He consulted me because of a history of myocardial illness, previous heart attack and subsequent coronary artery bypass surgery. His distress, which he thought was physical, was really emotional. He felt lonely and depressed in his marital relationship. After marrying for the first time at age 40, he had discovered that he had married an angry, hostile woman. Although his wife was attractive, he described her as being unavailable and unhappy. He experienced little passion with her and admitted to having sexual relations approximately once every three to four weeks. Although he wanted to break free from the relationship and was seriously considering separation, his fear of loneliness kept him trapped and stuck. He also did not want to leave his five-year-old son with whom he had a vital connection.

As we talked in subsequent meetings, I learned that he was always a little afraid of his wife and that she had dominated the entire relationship. I also learned that he had lost his mother at age three and that the dominant figure in his childhood home had been his older sister who in essence took the position of the mother. Since the loss of his mother must have created feelings of tremendous abandonment, he was not able to have any negative feelings toward his sister for fear of his sister leaving him. Consequently, he was trapped as a little boy in not experiencing his real feelings and later, he became trapped as an adult by the inability to leave his wife.

Inspired by an unconscious drive to find unconditional love and to establish a vital connection, he entered the clergy as a young adult. Fate intervened, for at age 30 he met a woman and had sexual relations for the first time. At age 33, he left the priesthood. John's father was very disappointed with this decision and once again, John experienced failure and the energy of rejection.

To overcome these feelings, John went to graduate school, earned a Ph.D. degree and became a college professor. After five years of a bad marriage, he suffered a massive myocardial infarction. After recovering from subsequent coronary artery bypass surgery, he was very disappointed that his older sister did not visit him. He had tremendous feelings of longing to visit his older sister but he was also afraid that she would reject him. His earlier childhood "stuff" came back to haunt him. The issues of heartbreak with the death of his mother led to tremendous vulnerability and fear of love resulting from the ultimate fear of abandonment. Such developmental issues of heartbreak, fear of love, threat of failure and fear of rejection set the stage for struggle which in itself is cardiac stress.

John's body reflected his feelings of deep sadness and unreleased anger. His eyes were swollen, narrow and listless. He spoke in a soft, sad voice and his look had very little conviction. His shoulders were rounded and his back was up and coiled, as if he was ready to attack in a fit of rage. This anger and resentment towards women was held in the upper torso of his body. It appeared that he was ready to strike out at any moment. When a child's relationship with his mother turns sour because he feels rejected, not understood, not seen, not loved, he cannot turn to another "mother." The inability to have angry negative feelings toward his older sister who took the place of his mother left John with considerable guilt which was expressed in his heart and sexuality; that is, he could not fully give to his wife. He could not surrender and be swept away. He needed to be in control of his feelings and would not allow his heart to be touched. His love could not be expressed with full conviction. His chest was armored and his heart was encased in a vise as if it were protected by a heavily armored shield.

The conflict in which John found himself was an unbearable

stress on his heart. Is John, therefore, vulnerable to heart attack? The answer is yes, but it does not mean that he will have another one. He is in a situation of great stress, but fortunately, he is free from other stresses. He is also able to cry and release feelings. He was willing to be soft, express his feelings and openly discuss his anguish. The experience of John's loss of love in his childhood was devastating. The experience of that loss was heartbreaking. Unfortunately, this happens to many children of our culture because many children are divorced from their parents in both the physical and emotional sense. The fear that opening one's heart to love could result in another experience of rejection and loss leads to a defensive attitude. We will see in a subsequent analysis how an individual armors against the threat of hurt and the possible pain of future heartbreak. It is the armoring process and rigidification of the chest wall which imposes a chronic stress upon the heart, eventually resulting in heart disease.

The stress of losing a loved one by death, divorce or breakup of a relationship can be so strong that it can trigger a fatal heart attack. There are many cases on record that attest to the fact that sudden cardiac death has occurred to persons upon learning of such a loss. The case of Alan, a 34-year-old male, comes to mind when discussing the circumstances of a near-fatal heart attack that he suffered on his birthday.

Alan had an unusual heart attack. When he arrived at the hospital, he was being resuscitated for sudden cardiac death. He was immediately taken to the cardiac catheterization laboratory. He underwent coronary arteriography, which outlines the circulatory system around the heart. He had no blockages, plaques or clogging of the vessels. No high-grade obstructions were present as one would see in individuals undergoing vascularization or coronary artery bypass. Alan's coronary vasculature just clotted; that is, his coronary arteries occluded and in the cardiac laboratory clots were being pulled out of his arteries through special types of catheters. Additional history indicated that he was of low risk. His serum cholesterol was 150. He had no history of diabetes or hypertension nor was he a smoker. He did have a positive family history of myocardial infarction (heart attack).

Since Alan was frustrated in not finding the reasons behind his heart attack, he consulted me. Alan had a myocardial infarction on his birthday. As he woke up that day, he had great expectations— after all, it was his birthday. After he went to work, he realized that his place of business had been broken into. It was not so much that equipment was missing, but rather the fact that his sophisticated alarm system had failed. He told me it was an incredibly stressful day. On a scale of one to ten it was a ten on that near fatal day. It was the worst day of his life. In the midst of tremendous stress over the burglary, he received a phone call from his girlfriend terminating their relationship. He thought that this was a very good relationship, but obviously it wasn't. After receiving the "Dear John" telephone call, Alan collapsed and was rushed to the emergency room. He was found to be in "ventricular tachycardia" and as he was undergoing CPR for minutes, he was shocked several times to restore his normal electrocardiographic rhythm. He was in and out of consciousness. I asked him several times what he was thinking about as he was on the verge of life and death and he told me that his girlfriend was in his thoughts. The heartbreak was incredible. Since his heart was telling the truth, it was running wild in a panic with ventricular arrhythmia. After he survived, he had tremendous feelings of despair and depression. In our interview, he told me that he felt powerless, but he did not get angry. I asked him why he did not get angry and he told me that he does not experience those feelings. Rather than experience his real self, he just held his feelings in. Even as we spoke, I had the sense that he was like a melon ready to burst in the sun with feelings and emotions, but he just held them in.

I asked him about his family. He stated that he was the second of five boys and had a very domineering and rigid mother. As we talked about her, some feeling started to emerge. He had considerable negativity toward his mother. Soon he told me about a movie he had seen a few weeks prior to his cardiac arrest. It was a movie that he did not like. It had a lot of sexuality and brutality in it. His mother kept telling him that he would like this production. Then she told him that he shouldn't have these feelings about the content and the performance. She kept on saying "you should, you should, you should" and he felt his whole body tighten and he just wanted to explode. He could never do that as a child and he couldn't do it now. He just held on to his feelings. As we talked, his breathing was contracted and shallow. He did not have any full respirations. He was breathing only very slightly and his chest was barely moving. There was no extension of the diaphragm. The breathing was lifeless. He had tension in his jaw. Although he smiled a lot in the interview, his smile was obviously a coverup for his anger. He did not want me to know that there was any anger in him. His back was hunched up and his shoulders were rounded, as if he were a cat ready to strike. I asked him if he was aware of how much anger he held and he said "I am aware of it, but I can't get it out". He never had support for such feelings. As we spoke for a while, I realized that I was dealing with a very contracted individual that was trapped in his own body. He also was covering up fear, but he did not want me to see that either. He really did not want me to see that he was experiencing any feeling whatsoever. In fact, I had the feeling that it was as if I were his parent. In other words, he tried to talk and explain everything. He was in his head and not experiencing his body. He was trying to convince me by his verbal expressions. He was really doing to me what was done to him as a child. He had this incredible urgency to get everything out as he tried to explain and rationalize. I realized on a body level that there was nothing there. His life was in his head. There was no feeling from the neck down.

Then he asked me what he could do to help himself. As we spent the afternoon together, I told him that he needed to be in therapy to work on his breathing, his held-in rage, and his heartbreak. He needed to experience feelings and he needed to reconnect with his girlfriend or establish a new connection. He also needed a spiritual connection and we talked about his going back to the synagogue and grounding in his roots. As we talked, we realized that his heart attack was really a new beginning. Alan's heartbreak was a manifestation of "not being seen." This was a reenactment of his childhood, which was later projected onto his girlfriend; that is, he unconsciously had tremendous longing to establish a deep feeling connection with his mother. With the loss of the girlfriend, he experienced the loss of another vital connection. His heart was under attack.

The loss of a loved one, either physically or emotionally can cause heartbreak. The loss or inability to make a vital connection with another person can also lead to unbearable loneliness evidenced by physiological changes that can be deadly. This experience of heartbreak is not uncommon among young children. The lost love is always that of the parent, putting the child in a very difficult position since he or she cannot make a new immediate connection to another parent. Crying, the earliest vehicle for maintaining connection between mother and infant, proves to be of no avail, so the child must adapt or give in to the loss and the pain. Adaptation is possible only if the pain can be suppressed and this is done by immobilizing the chest. This is a physical defense against the pain of lost love. This occurs when the individual fails to expire freely. Feeling is most acute as the chest softens at the end of respiration. Instead, the patient develops a type of denial that Reich called "inspiratory attitude." This defense takes the form of immobilization and the rigidification of the chest wall in denial of the loss. However, rigidity, as a form of defense, becomes a primary mechanism for the unconscious suppression of feeling.

Rigidity results from chronic muscular tensions in the voluntary musculature of the body, especially in the chest wall, neck and pelvis. Expression becomes limited as more impulses become blocked. Chronic spasticities and further tension develop. Segments of the body tend to become immobilized. Crying, expressing emotion and having feelings are stifled. Over time, such suppression of feelings and rigidification can extend throughout the depths of the organism including one's core involving the heart and lungs. For example, rigidification of the respiratory tree may result in asthma and/or bronchitis. Rigidification of the coronary vessels can result in the restriction of blood, thus making it harder for blood to reach the walls of the heart. Thus, a rigid defense in itself will become a chronic negative factor in the body creating a condition of muscular tension and limiting respirations. This is a profound cardiac stress. The immobilization of the chest wall is accompanied by tensing or contracting the muscles of the chest wall. Since it doesn't hurt anymore, the child can accept the loss of love. In time, the memory of the loss will be repressed and the adjustment complete. The heart, however, remembers.

CHAPTER 3

Mind, Body and Heart

Since ancient times the heart has been considered the pulsating source of life.

- In the 26th century B.C. the Yellow Emperor of China, Huang Ti, wrote, "The heart is the root of life" and the source of the "versatility of the spiritual faculties." Recognizing its mechanical functions, he added that the heart "influences the face and fills the pulse with blood."
- The Aztec sun worshipers linked the heart to the sun in their sacrificial ceremonies. The still-quivering heart of the victim was offered to the Sun to insure the protection and survival of their crops. In short, the heart and the sun were joined both in the symbolism and in the reality of their lives.
- The Bible has nearly a thousand references to the heart. The connection of heart and spirit is reflected in Psalm 51: "Create in me a clean heart, Oh God, and renew a right spirit within me." Many of my patients have gained tremendous strength from meditating on this one verse alone.
- "Late in the 19th century Kipling wrote in the "Recessional": "Still stands Thine ancient Sacrifice, an humble and a contrite heart." Here the heart is joined with the virtues of humility and contrition.

So who is man and what is the heart? Symbolically and poetically, the heart represents the very spirit, the core of the person, whether good or evil. In Genesis and in Jeremiah, the heart of man is described as evil. Our language is full of references to the heart and the nature of man. We may be described as open-hearted or closed, big-hearted or small, heavy-hearted or light-hearted, full of grief or joy. We may be lion-hearted or chicken-hearted. In love, we are said to give our hearts away. Others may "wear their hearts on their sleeves" being openly vulnerable to almost anyone or anything. When heart-broken, we may become cold-hearted. Hearts may jump or leap with joy or fall with disappointment. Our hearts may be shattered or strengthened. We may give up our hearts in despair or hope may raise our hearts. Our Valentines symbolize the heart as beloved. As Sextus Propertius declared around the time of Christ, "Absence makes the heart grow fonder." But beware, as Yeats says, "Too long a sacrifice can make a stone of the heart."

It may seem that all emotions and feelings are reflected into and felt in the heart and in the chest cavity where it is contained. To better understand how the heart plays such a pivotal role in our emotional and spiritual life, let us look at the complex internal communication system of man, the nervous system and the brain.

The Brain and the Heart

The nervous system is so vast and intricate, innervating and controlling every organ of the body, that it is descriptively divided in many ways. For our purposes, the most significant division is between the voluntary and involuntary nervous systems. This, however, is more a functional division than an anatomical one.

The voluntary nervous system describes those functions of

the body that are under our conscious control. The involuntary or autonomic nervous system, which is not under our conscious control, includes the major part by far of our nervous system and functions. Were this not so, we would be like the centipede trying to tell each leg where to go. Many of our functions such as breathing, for example, run automatically unless we consciously take charge of them. Even performing highly complicated procedures such as driving a car can be run "on automatic," allowing us to daydream or make plans for an upcoming meeting. Our involuntary functions, or those which are for the most part automatic, are sensitive to our emotions. When we are startled or frightened, for example, the diaphragm, our main breathing muscle, automatically flattens (inhales) and then stays flattened until the emergency is over and we exhale a "sigh of relief." Unfortunately, this is also true with chronic anxiety. Persons suffering from anxiety as well as those who have chronic respiratory disease or even women in labor are taught to take voluntary control of their diaphragm, inhaling, sighing or humming to promote exhalation.

The heart is even more vulnerable to our emotions. Only those far advanced in yoga or biofeedback can alter their pulse rate or blood pressure under experimental conditions and probably much less so under living stress. The heart, along with every other organ and system within the body, is not simply under the control of our emotions, but works within a system of checks and balances called homeostasis. First recognized by Walter B. Cannon, homeostasis is the body's ability to regulate itself by adapting to a particular environment, such as the way Eskimos develop more layers of internal body fat to protect against the cold.

Every force in nature is balanced by at least one and usually several forces. Our body temperature, for example, can be maintained within a span of something less than five degrees Fahrenheit, unless we are freezing to death or burning up with fever. It is only when we are sick or under severe physical or psychological stress that our bodies exceed the bounds of normal homeostasis.

Our emotions affect the heart through our endocrine glands and through the autonomic nervous system, which is divided into almost antithetical branches, the sympathetic and the parasympathetic systems. The sympathetic system prepares us for fight or flight whereas the parasympathetic accompanies relaxation, expansion and good digestion. The parasympathetic lowers pulse rate and pressure, stimulates the gastrointestinal movements and absorption, whereas the sympathetic increases heart rate and cardiac contraction while suppressing peristalsis and digestion. Therefore, when suddenly called for, most of the blood supply is directed to the brain and the musculoskeletal system.

Ancient man as well as modern man relied on the sympathetic nervous system for extra energy in situations of physical and emotional stress, athletic events or even combat. But such high arousal without an outlet for expression can be damaging. For example, we know that such emotional and psychological arousal can generate cardiac arrhythmias and coronary artery spasm, increase blood pressure, even provoke heart attacks and sudden cardiac death. What life-and-death communications travel between our nervous system and our heart? How can they produce such physiological and pathological responses to both real and sometimes imagined events?

The intricate relationship between the heart and the mind may be seen in the following case.

Larry, an ex-Marine, sustained a massive heart attack at age 37. Animated by large amounts of energy and drive, he worked at three jobs. He was clearly a Type-A personality, a typical candidate for a coronary. Larry was an aggressive overperformer and overachiever. Typically, he had little time or capacity for intimacy and pleasure. After Larry recovered from his heart attack, several studies showed the amount of heart damage he sustained. One study was a coronary arteriogram that demonstrated a total blockage of one of Larry's major coronary blood vessels accompanied by a swelling of the heart muscle. Physicians call this a ventricular aneurysm.

After the cardiac catheterization was finished, I asked Larry if we could investigate the emotional and/or mental side of his personality. He knew I was a psychotherapist and had a considerable interest in the intricate connection between the mind and the body. During this phase of the cardiac catheterization, a catheter was placed once again in Larry's heart. He was asked to think about past imagined stressful situations. He was asked to perform mental arithmetic and talk out loud. These were various interventions to see if the pressures inside Larry's heart would change with verbal communications or thinking about his previous Marine training or combat situations. Such an analysis would help determine if Larry's mind could effect intracardiac pressures within the confines of the left ventricle. During this evaluation, Larry was very cool and calm. The pressure in his heart did not seem to be significantly altered by any significant past stressful events or performing any mental arithmetic. Larry passed the test with flying colors, which demonstrated that his mind had little effect upon his circulatory system. He was a "cool cat" on the outside as well as the inside. His body was in harmony and free of any physiological imbalances. The pressure inside his heart was only slightly elevated which is expected in anyone who has suffered a heart attack.

During the next phase of the experiment, the catheter was again placed in Larry's heart and then I showed him his own coronary angiogram on videotape. When Larry saw the total occlusion of one vessel and a large swelling of his heart, he immediately imagined the strong possibility of follow-up reconstructive heart surgery. On the outside, Larry still looked cool. Although he appeared somewhat anxious to me, he continued to communicate that everything was okay. The computerized pressures, however, told the truth. Larry's intracardiac pressure increased by over 100 percent. In a few moments of visualization, this ex-Marine's exaggerated response to stress resulted in an overwhelming elevation of his heart's pressure; his altered self-perception induced a fight/flight response with secondary increase in adrenal-like neurotransmitters resulting in further deterioration of a heart that was already impaired.

When Larry thought about having surgery, he perceived a situation in which he would be helpless. This sense of helplessness triggered such a strong response that it presented a danger to his heart. Although Larry was totally unaware of his fear, i.e., denial, his alarm reaction or "overpreparedness" distinctly increased his cardiac vulnerability. It is not so surprising to learn that Larry had suffered a near-fatal heart attack at a young age. He is clearly what cardiologists call a "hot reactor;" that is, he is completely out of touch with the sensations and feelings in his body.

"Hot reactors" are among the hidden potential victims of cardiovascular disease. They are ordinary people who are out of touch or don't recognize or understand the messages their body is sending them. Their bodies gear them for battle when there is only a skirmish expected. Physiological overreactivity is yet another risk factor which goes beyond Type-A behavior. Clinical research suggests that consistent overreactivity precedes the development of hypertension and/or future cardiac events like a heart attack. "Hot reactors" are individuals who cannot tolerate uncertainty, loss of control or helplessness. In a crisis, they act and react. Larry was cool when he wasn't helpless, but when he watched his damaged and vulnerable heart, he experienced an immediate loss of control and his autonomic nervous system took over. This automatic response is typical in stressful situations for "hot" Type-A reactors. Let me examine further how his happens.

The Heart and the Autonomic Nervous System

Historically, the autonomic nervous system was thought to function independently of the central nervous system, thus it was thought to be autonomous. It is autonomous, but it is also part of a hierarchial involuntary nervous system of which the highest part belongs to the central nervous system. Without special experience or training, it is not under voluntary control.

Another name for the autonomic nervous system is the visceral nervous system; it controls the viscera (the internal organs) including the intestines, the glands, the heart and the smooth muscles of the blood vessels. It is also services our emergency responses and our emotions. These are not under voluntary control except as character traits, which we will discuss later.

As indicated in the previous section, the autonomic nervous system is divided into two complementary but oppositional branches, the sympathetic and the parasympathetic. Both are regulated by chemical messengers called neurotransmitters, rather than by neural impulses from the central nervous system. Remember that the parasympathetic works to conserve energy while the sympathetic enhances activity and stimulates responses to stress/danger or fight/flight by increasing the blood supply to the heart and skeletal muscles and decreasing the blood to the skin and the other organs.

The primitive autonomic nervous system, which lies entirely outside of the central nervous system (brain, brain stem and spinal cord), carries no conscious messages back to the central nervous system. It does, nonetheless, carry much vital information back to our central nervous system at the subcortical levels, specifically at the levels of the hypothalamus and the limbic system. We sometimes become aware of the effect of these messages when we begin to feel frightened, sad or angry without any obvious reason. Our heart may begin to race as some combination of information from our environment is being reflected in our own autonomic feeling-response. The autonomic nervous system is part of our sixth sense, an intuitive "gut feeling."

All emotions and most major reflexes can be contagious. If

someone yawns in a group, almost everyone in the group either yawns or has to stifle a yawn. The vomiting reflex is also very contagious. Have you every been on a rocky boat when someone becomes acutely sick? The nausea and vomiting spread rather quickly because of the reflex triggering of one's own fear of becoming ill. Fear is the most contagious of the emotions. For example, we have all heard of group hysteria such as the now-famous "soccer stampede" in England. To a lesser degree sadness is also transmissible. When someone cries at a funeral, it is a threat to the control system of almost everyone there. Love, on the other hand, is not based on fear and therefore is not contagious, although watching lovers makes us yearn for the vicarious feelings of warmth, comfort and connectedness. At the root of empathy is the autonomic system, although other systems of the CNS such as the visual, the proprioceptive and the kinesthetic also inform and affect our feelings of identity or repulsion to others.

The case of Larry clearly shows that the autonomic nervous system is under central control. Larry had only to imagine that his heart was damaged and that he might require surgery for his breathing to quicken and his internalized heart pressure to double. While the challenges of mental arithmetic and the revisualization of severe stresses that he had already survived left him unshaken in his confidence (his heart rate and pressure stayed well under control of normal homeostasis at rest), he had only to picture his damaged heart to "shake" him, making him even more vulnerable to cardiac events. If, on the other hand, Larry had been in touch with his fear and gave himself permission to express his fear through crying or even talking, this could have assuaged his condition. Thus, when the mind and body are connected, we have physiological balance. Our sympathetic nervous system works well when we are vulnerable and do not deny it. If, for example, we feel sudden, overwhelming sadness and allow ourselves to cry, this is healing to our heart. Anger works in much the same way when we are able to discharge the emotion in a grounded and positive way. Fear, the most visceral of all emotions, is under sympathetic control whether one is in denial or not. Ancient man fighting saber-tooth tigers relied on the fight-or-flight response of the sympathetic nervous system. For modern man, the sympathetic nervous system can be as equally important, but potentially destructive, as seen in the following analysis of "hormonal suicide."

Hormones and the Heart

The work of Walter B. Cannon, an American physiologist, encompasses a lifetime spent investigating sudden cardiac death, homeostasis and voodoo death. He used his term "fight or flight" to describe the functions of the sympathetic nervous system in acute stress. In his work with animals, he discovered and defined the function of the adrenalin-like hormones not only secreted by the sympathetic nerves, but also by the adrenal medulla, the core of the adrenal glands. These anger/anxiety hormones, adrenalin and noradrenalin, are released by such emotional circumstances as threat, uncertainty, danger and struggle. These are the struggle hormones that arise from defensive reactions to aggression, mobility and hostility. These hormones cause constriction of blood vessels, increase blood pressure, increase heart rate and cause various metabolic derangements such as an increase in cholesterol, free fatty acids and blood sugar, to mention a few.

Later, Hans Selye, the famous Canadian physiologist, made famous his theories of chronic stress. He described how the hormones of the adrenal cortex, the outer layer of the adrenal glands, secrete adrenal cortical hormones in response to our master gland, the pituitary. In turn, the pituitary is influenced by the hypothalamus, which is under the control of our limbic system and our cortex. This system, along with the sympathetic nervous system, is activated when stress is chronic.

When stress persists, as it often does for modern man, especially for those with certain personality and character traits, the abundance of cortisone-like hormones from the adrenal cortex begin to promote hardening of the arteries. This was shown in one particular study where excessive cortisol led to an increase in arteriosclerotic blockages of the coronary arteries. Vigilance or being constantly on guard (that sense of waiting for the other shoe to drop) may create an overabundance of cortisone, thus turning a psychological coronary risk factor into a physical one. With chronic vigilance, we can overdose on our own cortical and adrenal-like hormones, making the heart vulnerable to unexpected cardiac events such as heart attack, arrhythmia or even sudden death. It should be emphasized that this damage does not always occur immediately, but may occur when the adrenal glands are pushed to the point of exhaustion. Overwork, overstress and exhaustion, commonly called "burnout," are harbingers of death by hormonal overdose. Selye calls this the generalized adaptation syndrome.

Perhaps modern man is under more stress than the caveman because his adaptive responses were largely physical, whereas modern man does not usually indulge in physical responses. We have to keep cool and "fight back" mentally, leaving the nervous and cardiovascular systems in continuous overpreparedness and readiness. It is this continual state of visceral vascular readiness that makes the heart so vulnerable. For example, sophisticated clinical studies utilizing ambulatory monitoring devices have detected silent myocardial ischemia during the everyday psychological stresses of disagreements and confrontation.

Silent myocardial ischemia is a major risk factor for the heart. Myocardial ischemia can be defined as reduced blood flow to an area of the heart muscle due to a blockage of the

coronary arteries. It causes symptoms of chest pain or shortness of breath. Silent myocardial ischemia occurs when you
experience chest pain or shortness of breath but you don't
realize it. You may experience some feeling of discomfort but
you do not connect that discomfort to the heart or you may
feel absolutely nothing at all.

There are many people who have had this experience and
have been surprised when learning that their EKG revealed
the truth. I had one patient who said, "It was just a soft
little discomfort below my left shoulder blade" with her EKG
showing that her heart was in jeopardy. Another patient
stated, "I had discomfort in my left elbow" after his EKG
showed that he had coronary artery disease. Although silent
myocardial ischemia may occur in everyday situations like
driving or eating, it does occur more frequently in situations
of stress.

Other people truly may not feel the pain of their symptoms
because they are living in denial, which is a state of being cut
off from the awareness of what is happening to your body.
Living in denial, out of touch with your body and its feelings,
can lead to disaster. It can lead you to fail to admit that a
problem exists and to believe your symptoms are something
else. I have seen this situation in many excessively driven coronary-prone patients who have told me they thought they
were experiencing indigestion when in fact that were having
a heart attack. This kind of denial is also a major risk factor
for coronary artery disease. But is it denial or unrelieved stress
that causes the problem?

Along with another physician and psychotherapist, I created
my own study on unreleased stress and its relationship to illness. In a group therapy setting, participants were asked to
focus on their emotions, particularly on their feelings toward
unsatisfactory life situations, such as bad relationships, parental
conflicts and job stresses. Through measuring amounts of cortisone (the worry hormone) byproducts in the urine, we learned
that stress was a major factor in the production of the cortisol-

adrenalin-like hormones. Those in the group who expressed their feelings easily had average amounts of urine breakdown products. Those who admittedly held in their emotions had exceedingly high hormonal levels of cortisone in the urine. Interestingly, of the 24 people easily influenced by stress and unreleased emotion, five were men. And of these five, four had heart disease! These men refused to express their feelings during the weekend workshop and told me they preferred to "build walls around themselves" and to live in a "macho way" rather than to display sadness, especially through expressing feeling. These men were living in absolute denial of their stress. Denial is such an important cardiac risk factor that I will spend more time on it later in this chapter.

Selye confirmed this as well. His studies demonstrated that unrelieved stress led to increased levels of heart disease, hypertension, arteriosclerosis as well as diabetes and many other common diseases. Obviously we need a mechanism to help us learn to live with unrelieved stress. Crying, as previously stated, is one such way but there are others such as deep breathing, physical activity, releasing anger, talking about true feelings, having loving connections and sexual orgasms, to mention a few.

Pleasure is another way to combat stress. However when I ask many of my heart patients what they do for pleasure, I frequently get a typical "head answer" like "play with my computer," "read a book," "watch TV," etc. Many of us really do not connect with the pleasurable sensations of the body. Lowen, like Reich, feels that modern man is most afraid of pleasure. Even the simple bodily pleasures of life such as yawning or laughing, which often come unbidden and spontaneously, can be distressing. We see this in modern society when one stifles a laugh in a crowd, or when one needs to cover a yawn with the hand. If we inhibit such naturally innocent responses, it is no wonder that for many the sexual orgasm is repressed.

In bioenergetics, orgasm is described not simply as an ejaculation or a contraction of the uterus and vagina, but as a total body experience. This includes pleasurable streamings and convulsive movements that accompany the actual loss of genital sensation as the energy that was concentrated in the genitals and pelvis returns to other parts of the body in the climax. These streamings can also be felt in therapeutic massage. Here again we can see how pleasure may be inhibited if one cannot give oneself permission to emit even a release of feelings such as joy, crying or sadness. Massage, like other body-oriented therapies, may bring up old memories or feelings that have been stifled through chronic muscular armoring or tension. Such self-containment in expression is typical of the cardiac patient.

We can begin to see that the person who is chronically under the dominion of the sympathetic nervous system is often crippled. Relaxation is difficult because to relax is to let go of control, and to let go of control is at the very least to release a sigh and to feel something like a shiver or a streaming. To sustain any feeling would be a step in the right direction, but this is often not the case. Pleasure and feeling, often denied, are under the control of the will or ego. To control, to perform or to be the best is, unfortunately, a way of life. In his book *Narcissism, the Denial of Feeling*, Lowen tells us that narcissistic individuals breed narcissistic cultures that have become literally the insanity of our times. Such behavior focusing on performance takes us into our head and out of our body. This negates almost all general feeling and with it, pleasurable sensations as well.

Men like Larry, the ex-Marine discussed earlier, are usually very competent in bed. They hold erections a long time, but sometimes have difficulty in reaching a climax. Often they gain very little pleasure in their own bodies or in their release. Instead, they get the ego satisfaction of pleasing the woman, sometimes time after time. They are often known as "studs," and among their male companions, reveal their contempt for the women whom they serve.

The late Dr. John Bellis told me about another ex-Marine infantry sergeant, named Harry. He served with great distinction in Korea. He came to enjoy killing there and had to search for something in civilian life that could give him equivalent pleasure. He found it in killing sharks with a knife. Nothing compared with this, he said, certainly not sex! He must have been referring to what some call an "adrenalin rush." Harry's pleasure, and to varying degrees that of other Type A's, is sympathetic. It is the rush of the gambler, the daredevil, the race car driver and the mountain climber. It is the rush of fear that they know they can handle; the rush of adrenal excitement.

Adrenalin rush is the antithesis of pulsation, the natural ebb and flow of life energy in cells, tissues and organs. Pulsation is the key ingredient for health, integrating the energetic quality of body and mind. With pulsation, the body and the mind work together as one rather than as two entities. Thus, the mind moves the body and the body speaks its mind. Such an integration creates a harmony and freedom in movement. Every type of stress produces a tension in the body. Chronic tensions may persist after provoking stress has been removed, which we sometimes see in massage when suppressed feelings can be released by the manipulation of the muscles. Chronic muscular tensions disturb emotional health by decreasing one's individual energy, restricting one's mobility and limiting self-expression. When the energetic flow of the body expands, movements are unrestricted, coordinated and graceful. There is a harmony and freedom in effortless movement. Ballet dancers have grace in movement. A thoroughbred and a swan are said to be graceful, as is a dog that barks with both its mouth and its tail. Since graceful movements are integrated, the energy is not blocked and the whole organism flows. Grace is not connected nor directed; it is not willed; it is not related to drive or struggle. One cannot be graceful in struggling if the ego is involved. Such free-flowing movement with total involvement of the organism is seen in the pulsating quality of love.

I remember being in a workshop in Greece where I met a couple from Sweden. They were "in love." Although the woman, Margarita, was very pretty, her beaming and vibrating energy made her radiant and beautiful. And her smile gave it all away. Since she was so authentic, living in her heart and true self, I asked her for a definition of love. She came back with a swift reply: "Love is a feeling when every cell in your body vibrates." Vibration and pulsation together create core energy, which comes from the heart. In essence, the heart is where everything comes together, generating, for some, feelings of love, intimacy and tranquility; for others, fear and sadness; for still others, heartbreak and even heart disease. Being in love involves taking risks, being vulnerable, exposed and also daring to express one's deepest longings for true closeness and connectedness without pretense or masquerade. Again to quote Margarita, "Love is when the feelings become deeper, more mature and grounded. And yet, as we stand connected to the earth in our relationship, we touch the infinite of the great above and surges of energy buzz through our bodies. It is very moving."

On the other hand, disease can be seen in terms of energetic blocks where the organism's ability to pulsate in a particular body segment is stagnant or impeded. When an individual denies his or her infant and childhood emotions, the energy flow becomes distorted into physical and emotional blocks. Emotional blocks manifest in actual muscular rigidities that affect the body structure; this is called character armoring. Such blocks distort the person's functioning and reveal themselves in the way a person holds and moves his or her body. These spastic rigidities, the blocks of frozen energy, can eventually trigger organic disease. Such blocks in the chest, diaphragm and throat may render one susceptible to coronary artery disease.

Simply stated, if one has a block in breathing, one is not getting enough oxygen necessary for the healthy functioning of the heart. In many individuals with coronary artery disease, motility is disturbed and breathing is chaotic and not integrated. The normal pulsatory respiratory action becomes protracted and stagnant. Thus, the natural pulsatile flow of energy becomes disturbed. Such individuals, particularly men, have very little movement in their chest. This pattern has frequently been seen by nurses who take electrocardiograms. For example, when the electrodes are placed on one's chest, there is very little movement between inhalation and exhalation. Even though the patient is breathing, the electrodes appear to be still.

The breathing patterns of coronary-prone Type-A individuals has been studied in regard to inspiration and expiration. In one such study, the inspiration and expiration times for the coronary-prone, Type-A individual were considerably shorter than for a group of noncoronary-prone Type-B participants. When inhalation and exhalation are slower and nonchaotic, more oxygen exchange occurs in the lungs, thus giving the body a greater oxygen saturation. Previously, I told you about aggressive, coronary-prone individuals who suck in breath during speech even while continuing to speak and then exhale brief sighs and/or muffled grunts when breathing out. Such disturbance of respiration results in a charged, non-pulsating energetic cycle that consists of fixation on inhalation and mobilization during exhalation with subsequent difficulties in relaxation during the breathing cycle.

Free-flowing oxygen transference is often interrupted by the inability to breathe deeply. When one is healthy, one is fully alive in one's breathing and in one's body. Expansion, pulsation, and pleasure are thus in harmony. Such an individual is in contact with the environment and in contact with the self. This person is healthy and free of disease. This is pulsation. This is grace.

Chronic tension, on the other hand, occurs through trapping energy within the body. The inability to experience feelings renders individuals susceptible to heart disease. Now we can see the difficulty we face if we are to free ourselves of symptoms and diseases of heart and body. Healing a heart is not just a matter of manipulating risk factors, hormones or drugs, nor is it just a matter of changing habits and attitudes. Although these aspects are important in the healing process, getting well requires a mobilization of all our own intrinsic forces that offer resistance to disease. And, we must be willing to change patterns and lifestyle habits.

The cause of heart disease is multifactorial. Although the physical risk factor model is extremely important, the emotional side of heart disease is equally important, although frequently underestimated. The early framework of heart disease is not only the fear of love, but also the fear of healthy emotional expression. Just as fulfillment of love enhances the pulsatory or free expression of the child, the loss of love is devastating. Such childhood heartbreak may be caused by conditional love or lack of love and understanding from the parents. In conforming and being good, looking for love and acceptance, the child acts in accordance with parental desires and tries to avoid future heartbreak by not expressing real feelings. In the process of building defenses around his or her heart, the child shuts down and turns off needs—living in a false self. But such protection from the hurt of childhood becomes a future trap for heart disease in the adult. The armoring process that began in childhood rigidifies the chest wall and places an undue stress upon the heart by affecting the breathing pattern and, therefore, the natural pulsatile quality of the heart.

When one denies feelings, one denies one's heart. This betrayal of self is rooted in the survival techniques of childhood that we sometimes call character. The relationship of character to cardiac pathology is frequently entwined in a patient's fate. Such may be the case in the phenomenon of the Sudden Death Syndrome, which follows in the next chapter.

CHAPTER 4

―――∽――

Sudden Death

- A corporate executive on his way up in the company has found his expected promotion blocked due to company politics. It will come, but not as soon as he had anticipated. Meanwhile, his work goes on; he feels pressured, but no more so than usual. He has, however, begun to develop headaches and shortness of breath, both of which generally disappear on weekends. Life at home is pretty much the same; relationships are fine, if occasionally unsatisfactory. In the last month, however, he has had to buy a new car, pay for his son's braces and try to understand his wife's need for increased self-fulfillment. It is now Saturday evening and our executive is unwinding from his time-pressured, hectic week by having dinner in a local restaurant with his wife and another couple. Over cocktails and cigarettes, they laugh, sharing stories of family situations and job pressures. They order bottles of wine and enjoy a dinner high in fat and cholesterol content. Later that evening, our corporate executive suffers a massive fatal heart attack.
- After finishing her laundry, a woman in her mid 50's experiences some dizziness and slight sweating. After resting a few minutes, she begins to walk up the stairs, only to experience weakness and lightheadedness once again. Her breathing is labored and she lacks feeling in

69

her legs. She cannot feel her body, especially from the waist down. She is so weak that she could "drop." She needs to do the shopping, fold the clothes and prepare dinner for her husband and children. But, instead she, too, experiences sudden cardiac death.

- A man wakes in the morning feeling unwell and complains of pain and distress in his chest and abdominal area. He is sweating profusely and gasping for air. His alarmed wife calls 911, but before the paramedics arrive, the man expires.

Sudden cardiac death is the number-one killer of people in the 35-to-60 age group. This presents a major challenge to the contemporary cardiologist. Clinical studies have determined that from 10 to 40 percent of the time the first recognized symptom of heart disease is a fatal heart attack. This is not an unusual occurrence. The major problem with cardiac disease is that it happens with little or no warning. Although some afflicted individuals may have signs of coronary insufficiency, i.e. chest discomfort, shortness of breath, sweating or light-headedness, frequently there are no symptoms or warnings associated with heart illness. Heart disease is ominous in its silence. Ninety percent of individuals with heart disease are asymptomatic. Heart attack or sudden death is frequently the first sign of heart disease.

Do patients with heart disease really experience no symptoms or do they just ignore or deny them? Are ordinary people out of touch with their feelings and their bodies? Is it merely an inability to interpret the signals that the body sends the mind? For many, such is the case. But for others, there is a total denial of feeling from the neck down.

When patients come into my office, they are, for the most part having problems or symptoms. People will read off a shopping list of symptoms and ask me to diagnose their problem. Many patients will talk about this or that going on in their lives. Some will listen to their body signals, but many are completely out of touch; that is, the mind is saying one thing while the body is saying something different. Frequently, the most significant symptoms are not even communicated. Such a disconnection between the mind and the body is usually the result of denial. In the previous chapter I told you how denial can be a major cardiac risk factor. Let me illustrate this with the case of Jim.

In 1977, soon after completing my fellowship in cardiology, I went to the local bank to open a checking account for my new practice and dealt with a banker I will call Jim. About a month later, Jim appeared at the emergency room with a heart attack. Here is his story:

Jim was opening up a checking account for a new client just as he had done for me. He felt he had given the new client ample time to ask his many questions, but the client persisted with more questions and concerns. Since Jim had another client waiting, he was becoming "time urgent" and felt trapped.

Jim should have told his new client that he had an appointment with another client and that his time was up. But instead, he chose to withhold his emotions and frustrations. He was feeling so much stress that he actually had to wipe the sweat off his forehead.

Jim totally denied this body sensation as well as all the messages his body was sending him. His hands began to sweat, he had difficulty breathing, he became dizzy and developed chest pain.

Thinking that his pain was just "indigestion," Jim let no one know how he was truly feeling. Fifteen minutes later, he was brought to the emergency room with a heart attack.

Thus, a seemingly everyday occurrence ended in tragedy. But why? Why does a man put so much strain on his body that he ends up in total collapse? The answer is simple. Jim was living in denial.

Living with awareness about your body is really the key to

preventing ill health. Jim denied all the signals his body was sending him. He probably could have prevented his heart attack if he had only communicated his feelings, taken a few deep breaths, and told his client the truth. Instead, he pushed beyond his normal expectations and almost died in the process.

Jim, like many of my patients, was really out of touch with his body. He was not connected between the head and the body. He really did not listen to any of the conversations that went on between his brain and his heart.

Denial may take many forms. There can be physical, spiritual, emotional or especially mental expressions. For example, on the physical plane, one may not wish to listen to the body, as in the case of our typical corporate executive. He ignored and violated nearly all of the risk factors associated with heart disease; therefore his body paid for his lifestyle. Generally, the question is "Why?" Why does a person put so much strain on the body when the end result is bound to be illness? The answer, complicated and relative, lies in the needs that are misinterpreted, fears that are unspoken and a will to succeed according to others' and society's standards. To begin to alter this uneven struggle between needs and will is a lifelong task. To live up to this false and perfect image requires a lot of energy; thus stress in the end can be self-destructive. For these individuals, the question is not so much "why," as "how?" How can they maintain their goals, meet their ego needs and yet keep their bodies from paying too high a price? The answer is woven into the word "denial," six letters that have become the literal executioner of the whys and hows or even of life itself.

On a spiritual level, denial manifests itself in the false belief of physical indestructibility.

Another patient of mine is Bill, a 45-year-old oil and gas executive with a history of cardiomyopathy. The cause of his heart disease was unknown. He had undergone a cardiac catheterization and myocardial biopsy which demonstrated fibrosis of his myocardial fibers and a large, poorly-functioning heart muscle. His arteries were fine and free of disease, but his heart muscle was deteriorating. Bill was an athlete in high school and in college. He had a real love for sports and activities. After coming down with heart disease he continued to deny the significance of his illness; that is, he continued to drink alcohol, follow an imprudent diet and pursue activities he was barely capable of performing. He acted as if he were immortal. After all, he was a senior vice president of a large corporation, was making lots of money and had tremendous self esteem. He had over 200 employees under his supervision and management. He was an "important" strong man. Why shouldn't he consider himself immortal? In living up to his image, he covered up his weak and deteriorating heart. By being in a false self, he acted as if he didn't have a heart problem.

I remember the week before Bill died. Since his myocardial function was severely compromised, we talked about moderation. I advised him again about the perils of overeating, overdrinking, overworking and even overexercising. Superficially, he appeared to take in my recommendations; however, his unconscious drive to sustain his image was stronger than the wish to comply with good advice. He was driven and determined to do as he wished. The day he died, he went on a five-mile bike ride. After the strenuous exercise, he was exhausted, had a couple of cold beers, went to bed and never woke up.

Like General George Armstrong Custer leading his 7th Cavalry into the Valley of Little Bighorn, Bill's belief in his false powers was really a denial of his vulnerability. For Custer, it was the denial of the possibility of a superior force more robust than the 7th. For Bill, it was the denial that his heart could win out over his head. Custer recklessly imposed his will to succeed at all costs, hoping victory would enable him to become the next president of the United States. Bill's desire was to live in his image of the powerful CEO. Both met their fate by exercising their wills.

Such misuse of willpower may also be related to the unconscious fear of expansion; that is, unknowingly overstepping one's boundaries, thus inviting failure or even death. I remember one individual who was at the Saratoga Race Track only a couple of hours before having a heart attack. He had just won a great amount of money and came to our emergency room with chest pain and shortness of breath. The look on his face was one of fear, doom and hopelessness. As he was being placed on a stretcher and his garments removed, the nurses commented on how much money he had in his pockets. I don't know the exact amount, but this man had hundreds of one hundred dollar bills in his wallet, pockets and trousers. I remember thinking at the time, too much money could be hazardous to your health!

While I had only a few minutes to take a history from this man, he told us he had won a large sum of money and became extremely excited. While I believe the man was genuinely happy, his excitement was really a cover-up of underlying tension, perhaps feeling that he was not worthy of the money, that he could lose the money or possibly even make more money. He continued betting despite the "indigestion" in his chest. He was short of breath, but disregarded that sensation too. My brief patient was totally out of touch with his feelings. After two or three more races, in an unbounded state, he collapsed and was brought to the emergency room at Albany Medical Center Hospital where, unfortunately, he expired one half-hour after arrival, regardless of our attempts to resuscitate him.

Why, you might ask, would a fatal heart attack occur in a seemingly very joyous situation? There are no easy answers in dealing with such manifestations of stress, but the key here is self-perception. Our successful bettor was on a roll. Refusing to recognize his physical discomfort, he continued betting, seeing himself as a "winner." However, he was out of touch with his body and therefore was in reality a "loser." Had he sought earlier medical attention, perhaps the outcome would have been different. Altered perceptions, or the mind saying one thing and the body revealing another, is really the essence of what cardiologists frequently call "silent myocardial ischemia" or when an EKG is telling us the heart is in trouble, but the patient has no sensation. More succinctly, the body is telling the truth as the heart is revealing its distress.

The major challenge for a contemporary cardiologist like myself is really assessing individuals at risk for sudden cardiac death. Most cardiologists, in general, know that denial is a big factor. Moreover, we frequently are overaggressive in the approach to diagnosing cardiovascular disease because we cannot just rely on a patient's story. Their statements are often fragmented, unclear and misleading. Patients really don't want to believe they could have a potentially fatal illness. This belief is expressed in their story which is sometimes a masquerade of the "real" problem.

Stress is really a disconnection between the brain (thinking) and the heart (feeling). This total negation of self, a frequent accompaniment of human nature, is particularly seen in aging men.

For example, many of my male patients with cardiac disease seem to think that retirement would be in their best interest. But for many, retirement is a death sentence. That is, when men retire and lose the purpose in their lives with the cessation of their job and productivity, they often die. Studies have shown that cardiovascular deaths among men increase dramatically in the first year of retirement. This scenario may also pertain to women. To sever the work connection also severs their real connections to life. Many men deny the importance a job plays in their lives and, of course, not all men die when they retire. Some men experience the retirement years as the most pleasurable and satisfying in their lives. Perhaps, however, these men have connections that are more vital than their work. Perhaps these men have loving relationships with their

spouses or significant others. These connections are healing
to the heart. In a study by a Russian gerontologist in the
Ukraine, 15,000 individuals over age 80 were examined in regard to longevity. Ingredients for a long life included the contin-
uation of working and sustaining loving, warm relationships.
There is nothing greater in life than intimacy, support and a vital
emotional connection to keep life worthwhile.

In our inquiry into denial, we know that the mind and
body can influence each other. To be in touch with the self
is to be in touch with the body and all its feelings. To be out
of touch and totally unaware may have serious effects as seen
in a study of marathon runners, seven of whom died suddenly
while running. At postmortem, it was discovered that many
of these individuals had severe coronary artery disease. In fact,
this illness is so ubiquitous and silent that it had occurred
unknowingly in these trained athletes. In cardiac illness, are
symptoms a poor indicator of disease or not? Could all these
marathon runners be asymptomatic? Or could they have
symptoms and be living in denial. That was the focus of the
analysis.

There is little warning for sudden death. It occurs frequently in young males and again without their knowledge,
about three-quarters of the victims have advanced coronary
artery disease. No one expects to become a sudden death sta-
tistic, yet of the nearly one million persons who die each year
from some form of cardiovascular disease, almost half will die
suddenly and unexpectedly. Sudden cardiac death, in most
cases, begins with a wild torrent of electrical impulses that
seriously disrupt the rhythm of the pulsating heart. Cardiologists refer to this as sustained malignant arrhythmia in which
the heart muscle twitches but doesn't adequately pump. But
what are the factors that contribute to such vulnerability?

Considerable clinical evidence now indicates that psychological or emotional stresses may trigger the development of
ventricular arrhythmia especially in individuals with impaired

coronary circulations. In general the terminal event is probably ventricular fibrillation, although in some cases sudden cessation of the heartbeat altogether may occur. Many subjects at autopsy have myocardial infarction, but at least 20 percent of the cases have no structural heart disease at all. This suggests that the fatal arrhythmia may have been provoked by some neurometabolic mechanism resulting from stress. This was probably the case in the famous sudden cardiac death of the English anatomist John Hunter who died suddenly during a heated argument proclaiming that, "My life is in the hands of any rascal that cares to annoy or tease me."

There is increasing evidence to support the view that a wide range of psychosocial factors and environmental influences such as depression, exhaustion, divorce, job loss and low socioeconomic status predispose us to neurogenic and neuroendocrine influences that may provoke a fatal cardiac disturbance. Over the course of time, stress-induced myocardial damage may promote malignant cardiac arrhythmia. From autopsy studies, small areas of patchy necrosis associated with scar formation are present in more than 80 percent of the hearts in victims of sudden cardiac death. These lesions are indistinguishable from such cardiac scars produced in animals by the administration of catecholamines (adrenalin-struggle hormone). Researchers suggest that these small patchy scars, produced by an overabundance of adrenalin, become the breeding ground for life-threatening ventricular arrhythmia.

We know, for example, that there are strong behavioral and psychological factors that frequently precipitate cardiac arrest. It is no coincidence that sudden psychological or emotional stress frequently occurs just prior to a cardiac event. What intrigues me about sudden death is why Monday is the most prevalent day of the sudden death occurrence. Approximately 36 percent of all sudden deaths occur on Mondays. The second leading day is Saturday. Why? Is it the result of psychologically and emotionally gearing up or gearing down for the week's activities? Is the office a safe place? Or is it a place of combat and stress for the heart? We can look at this both ways. Some people may loathe going to work and others may loathe going home. Wherever the stress is, the heart will reveal it and tell the truth.

Experimental research has demonstrated the impact of acute psychological stress on sudden cardiac death. In one study, 91 percent of the patients who experienced sudden cardiac death and who were successfully resuscitated related that they were experiencing acute psychological stress at the time of their sudden death experience. A typical scenario might be: a middle manager is winding down after a busy week. The economy is in a recession. He has to cut costs. His overhead is high. There is a potential of losing his job and with it, a loss of self-esteem. He is not involved in a loving relationship and is isolated and depressed. He is exercising at a health spa and suddenly hears some unexpected disturbing news. He experiences a sudden cardiac event.

Like acute psychological stress, chronic depression has also been known to be a factor in the sudden death syndrome. In a clinical evaluation of 54 patients with clinical depression, Green and colleagues determined that depressed individuals who suddenly experience an unpleasant event are more prone to sudden death. The problem is that depression, like cardiac disease, is also frequently silent and not recognized by the individual. If you ask a person if he is depressed, he will look at you in a strange way and say no. Many of my patients have told me that they are "not depressed." Again, this is coming from their heads and not their bodies. But if I ask them how they find pleasure in their lives, they frequently don't know or it's a mystery to them. Their sleep patterns are poor and sexuality is the furthest thing from their minds.

People will not tell you they are depressed. They will cover it up and deny it. They mask it. Loss of interest in their partners and a reluctance to get to know their children frequently occurs. For example, they do not have the energy to be interested in their child's athletic endeavors or their school work or even how they are feeling inside. They won't know or forget their partner's favorite color. They are so caught up in their inner struggle that they have little room for any awareness of others. But again, they will not tell you they are depressed. They lack aliveness and feeling and have no interest or spontaneity in everyday things. This is depression. Depression occurs when one denies heartbreak and in the process refuses to release it and grieve it. As a clinical cardiologist and psychotherapist, most depression I see is the result of the loss of or the threatened loss of vital connections.

Throughout life, we are constantly making connections, superficial to some and more deeply to others. By saying goodbye to the old and taking on the new, connections may have variable levels of feeling. For example, a warm personal relationship may have more depth of feeling than a connection to a job. The love for a child may have a different meaning than the love for a spouse. Such vital connections are those associations that affect one's core energy or the vitality of the organism. Loving vital connections induce expansion and enhance the natural ebb and flow or the natural rhythm of the heart. The loss of these vital connections may affect the health of the heart by causing chest pain or erratic contractions due to the shock of the loss. The loss of a vital connection can induce heartbreak and thereby affect the pulsating quality of the heart and the ultimate health of the person. Many of us have had the painful experience of deep hurt and anguish expressing itself in our hearts and chests.

Chest pain, arrhythmia and sudden shortness of breath are symptoms frequently associated with heartbreak. If one experiences the loss of a vital connection, one has a choice of either establishing a new connection or withdrawing into one's self. The latter frequently results in loneliness, isolation and depressive-like symptoms. If, however, the loss of a vital connection is balanced by establishing a new connection, the organism adapts. If a new connection cannot be established, the individual may be faced with a sense of doom and a loss of hope. This overwhelming feeling of despair sets up hormonal interactions between the mind and the body that can create feelings of panic, which in turn may lead to myocardial vulnerability and possibly ventricular fibrillation. Thus, in the sudden death sequence, the loss of a vital connection, i.e. a loved one, relationship, job or bodily function may result in a sense of doom and panic. If the organism cannot adapt, it must find a way to escape from the intolerable situation. Not infrequently, sudden death occurs. Although it is a "maladaptive escape," it is at least a way out of such hopelessness and despair.

I remember the unfortunate case of a 52-year-old diabetic woman who had spontaneously bled into her eye and required emergency surgery. Two years before, she had sustained a heart attack but had since been enjoying a good quality of life. She was not experiencing any symptoms of chest pain or shortness of breath. She was admitted to the hospital and underwent immediate surgery which, unfortunately, was unsuccessful. Upon learning of the loss of her eyesight, she became deeply saddened and depressed. I remember seeing her in the hospital ward and feeling her depth of sorrow. Sitting in a wheelchair, she was despondent that she couldn't see. She talked in a monotone voice and kept her head down. She said that she had lost all hope and had nothing to look forward to. She died one day later.

There are lethal conversations between the brain and the heart. These conversations are mediated through the nervous system by way of chemical messengers called hormones that serve as harbingers of death. Yes, we can overdose on our own body adrenalin in situations such as fear, horror, excessive arousal or deep despair and depression. The body can commit suicide by overstimulating the heart. Thus, the heart running wildly in a panic terminates in ventricular fibrillation.

In primitive societies, there is a syndrome called voodoo death, first researched in detail by Walter B. Cannon, who studied voodoo death in the islands of the Pacific, Australia and Africa. He tells us that voodoo death defies the imagination of Western man. For example, he reports accounts of warriors who die in battle, not from wounds but as a result of a witch doctor's curse, or rather, their belief in the inescapability of the curse. With such a belief in the supernatural, a common feature among the cursed is heightened emotional arousal. The possessed victim and the other members of his family or clan believe that he is doomed to die. The belief in black magic is societal. Since this is a cultural phenomenon, the doomed victim not only has to deal with the sheer unmitigated terror of the curse, but also he is physically isolated and literally ostracized from the rest of society. He is all alone in the struggle that eventually ends in death. But how and why does he die? Does the social isolation, intense loneliness and despair cause a loss of hope and a willingness to die? Or is it the curse itself? Many of these deaths are commonly preceded by alienation, isolation and lack of social support for the doomed victim. Cannon concluded that these solitary and insecure people were overcome by fear and terror without the safety net of a supportive environment. Therefore, they accepted death as a way to escape a miserable situation.

Still, this does not explain the physical mechanism of death. Cannon concluded that the overwhelming stimulation of the sympathetic nervous system resulted in the provocation of lethal electrical instability to the heart. In contemporary terms, doctors would describe the sudden death sequence as a result of malignant arrhythmia culminating in ventricular fibrillation. Acute coronary spasm and heart attack could be other possibilities. It is important to remember, however, that these deaths were precipitated by such a profound loss of hope that all attempts to revive these individuals were to no avail. Here again, we see that psychological belief can determine one's physical destiny.

Suicidal behavior is yet another example of the psychological overwhelming the physical. A case study during my internship comes to mind.

It was New Year's Eve in 1972. I was the psychiatrist on call at the Albany Medical Center Hospital. I had received a phone call at approximately 4 A.M. from the switchboard operator. She had a man on the line asking to talk to the "shrink" on duty. He told her that he had a gun and had threatened to kill himself. Although this event occurred more than 20 years ago, I do remember the pertinent elements in the conversation.

Although the conversation lasted for over two hours, I lacked a rapport with him. Something was missing. I specifically remember the turning point in the conversation when I finally made a connection with him. I was "an ear" and a nonjugmental voice for this stranger and I was honest and sincere in my remarks. He asked me many questions and I replied. When I talked about my personal life and my own struggles, he listened. At this point in the conversation, I felt we had established a sense of trust. After I found this opening, I made one simple clear statement about my feelings concerning suicide. It went something like this, "The problem with suicide is that you may want to kill yourself today, but maybe not tomorrow." After I made these comments, there was a pause in the conversation. The man listened and he was taking this in. His tone of voice changed. It was then I invited him to the emergency room and offered to help him. "I'll be there Doctor," he said and I replied, "I'll wait for you."

Minutes later, he came to the emergency room and was admitted voluntarily to our locked ward. Through treatment, I later learned my patient's major issue was the inability to take in help, especially from men. This was obviously a problem that he had had with his father which was eventually resolved through counseling. The patient was eventually discharged and a year later, he wrote me a letter to say he was doing well and was glad to be alive.

I am convinced my patient's survival depended upon the moment we connected and developed a trust. Now he had hope. In a critical moment of despair, any connection, no matter how simple or trivial, can change the course of events. Although it can occur in the flicker of a moment, it may be enough to prevent a suicide. Establishing a vital connection can indeed be lifesaving. On the other hand, the loss of connections or the perceived loss of all hope can be deadly. The siege at Stalingrad is such an example.

Hitler, like his predecessor Napoleon over 100 years before, made the fatal error of invading Russia, thus creating two fronts and dividing his forces. The Russian winter was brutal, unforgiving and deadly. Hitler's sixth and best army was to defend Stalingrad at all costs. Thousands of men were ordered to hold the position to the death. Although retreat would have saved hundred of thousands of soldiers' lives, this would have cost Hitler his image as a leader and would have forced him to acknowledge a mistake. Stalingrad will not go down in history as a site of ferocious combat, but rather as a death-ghetto resulting from political wartime propaganda. False messengers to Germany indicated that generals and privates were fighting side by side to the very last bullet. The German people were receiving this news, but it was not true. The truth of the matter was not that Stalingrad had become a siege but that men were dying slowly by exposure, cold and starvation. Although some soldiers died in combat, many deserted and most died of the unforgiving elements of nature. Many also ended their lives swiftly with self-inflicted wounds; Hitler's best Panzer troops were committing suicide. Here again, the mind, in a strange way, chose death as a way out of an agonizing situation. Since these men were not permitted to surrender, they lost all sense of hope, preferring a quick bullet to the head over a painful slow death.

The loss of hope is deadly. One can either voluntarily pull the trigger or involuntarily die of heartbreak or some other maladaptive disease. Both ways, however, terminate an individual's life.

Loss of hope, heartbreak, despair, intense loneliness and the loss of vital connection affect not only the vitality and the health of the organism, but also its destiny. But are there ways to protect ourselves in such overwhelming and undesirable life situations? The answer is yes. Love is the most powerful of all emotions and holds the answer to man's search for comfort.

Many of us have heard stories of survivors or testimonies of people overcoming ordeals against great odds. Probably the most extraordinary circumstances of survival would include the death camps of World War II. Concentration camp survivor and psychiatrist Victor Frankel states that under these circumstances we need to find meaning in suffering. In his book, *Man's Search for Meaning*, Frankel reports a mystical and spiritual experience that he had as a prisoner. In such a spiritual moment, he was able to retreat from the terrible surroundings to an inner freedom of love and joy. On one morning during a cold March day, as he was stumbling in the darkness awaiting a kick or the butt of a rifle, spontaneous thoughts of his wife came to mind. In a moment of grace, of physical and spiritual oneness with the universe, he imagined his wife with uncanny awareness. He had a visual and auditory experience of her. And as he thought about her, his mind dwelled on a universal truth. The truth is that, "Love is the ultimate and the highest goal to which a man can aspire." Frankel continues:

Then I grasped the meaning of the greatest secret that human poetry and human thought and belief have to impart; the salvation of man is through love and in love. I understood how a man with nothing left in this world still may know bliss, be it only for a brief moment, in the contemplation of his beloved. In a position of utter desolation, when man cannot express himself in positive action, when his only achievement may consist in enduring his sufferings in the right way—an honorable way—in such a position, man can, through love and contemplation of the image he carries of his beloved, achieve fulfillment.

Frankel then goes on to say that love goes beyond the physical person of the beloved and finds its deepest meaning in its spiritual being and in one's inner self. Here again, we see that love is the cardinal motivating factor in survival.

But not all of us have the good fortune to experience true love of another, or of self for that matter. In its absence, is there anything else? Are there other key elements we can rely on to protect ourselves in such intolerable and undesirable life situations? The answer is yes. My patients, again, have been my teachers. For example, I have been able to watch some of my patients rise above utterly hopeless situations through the power of another vital connection: faith. When all medical technology, pharmacological agents, devices, and heroic measures are exhausted, I have always resorted to the phrase "hope and a prayer." The case of Mary illustrates the profound connection of hope, faith and love.

Mary was a woman in her late 50's who came into our hospital with intense abdominal pain. She had what doctors call an "acute abdomen" and underwent surgery to investigate the cause of her illness. At the time of surgery, she was found to have a gangrenous bowel as a result of occlusion of the central veins in her intestines. The medical terminology for such a condition is mesenteric thrombosis. The surgeons who performed the operation took out approximately two feet of inflamed bowel. After the initial successful surgery, the patient subsequently deteriorated and redeveloped abdominal pain and swelling. Because of her deterioration, she was operated on a second time. At this time, the doctors found extensive amounts of discolored bowel which was in jeopardy of becoming gangrenous. Because the surgeons could not remove all of her intestines, they closed her up and told me of the terminal and grave situation. At this time, massive doses of blood-thinning agents were utilized hoping to save the intestines. The patient was sent from the recovery room back to her room and eventually told of the unsuccessful results.

I remember speaking to her and her family. I explained the situation as grave but not hopeless. I specifically told them that a large section of her intestines was in jeopardy of necrosis or cell death. In such a seemingly hopeless situation, I offered them all the medical technology that was available, such as antibiotics and blood thinning agents. I ended my comments with hope and optimism.

In my mind, I knew the situation was probably terminal, but not hopeless. When speaking to the family and patient I recommended hope and prayer. What I didn't realize, however, was that this was a very religious family and the patient had a strong faith in God. The family notified perhaps 100 churches all over the state of Connecticut. I was told by her relatives that literally hundreds of thousands of people were praying for Mary. Mary believed that she would get well because of her strong belief and faith. A few days later, she actually began to improve. After approximately one-and-a-half weeks, she was taking nutrition by mouth and after four weeks, she walked out of the hospital. Was it a miracle that saved this woman? Or was it her own belief that she could be saved?

Just as a victim of the voodoo curse believes in the overwhelming suggestion of darkness and death, Mary had no doubt that all the support and prayer would save her. The voodoo victim is ostracized, lonely and despondent. Mary was supported, nurtured and overwhelmingly hopeful. Both were believers: one in death and one in life. Mary had the belief that God would save her and she survived.

As a doctor, I have learned that one's belief in getting well is perhaps the greatest element in healing. The doctor should

never take away the feeling of hope. Hope is essential to healing and survival. During my medical student days, I remember
one of my professors at Albany Medical Center (a cancer
hospital) telling us that as a physician, we should never take
away a patient's hope. Even with patients diagnosed with cancer and heart disease, it is imperative to encourage them to
make future plans, buy new clothes, plan a vacation and cele-
brate birthdays and holidays. I remember telling one patient
with terminal heart failure that his next scheduled appointment was going to be in three months. He looked at me and
asked, me, "Do you think I'll make it?" I looked at him eye
to eye and told him he would. He was in my office three
months later and to this day is still a viable patient in my
practice. He is one of many who has a future. Caring physicians will always give their patients hope, since having hope
keeps the future alive.

In the Bible, Paul states in the letter to the Corinthians that
the three greatest emotions are faith, hope and love, of which
love is the most enduring. Trite as this may sound, these are
the essentials. These are the gifts, the real arts of healing, that
frequently must be utilized in a doctor/patient relationship.
Paul's letter to the Corinthians has often spoken to my own
heart and it has been a reminder of the essential and meaningful core feelings of life.

In my experience as a cardiologist and a psychotherapist, I
have coached many of my patients in experiencing feeling. I
asked them to express their feelings, to be real, to be authentic,
and most of all, to be true to themselves. Channeled correctly,
the emotions and reactions that hurt the body can also heal
it. The trick is to be able to look at something negative and
find some positive force, no matter how small; to be able to
laugh at oneself and not take everything quite so seriously; to
be able to communicate honestly and to be able to reach out,
love and, in return, accept the sincere affection of others.
These are the forces and positive emotions that heal. When

one lives authentically, that is, according to true feelings, one knows that good prevails over evil and that the truth always works. Such an intuitive knowing and a belief in the truth helped me get through a most heartbreaking ordeal.

In 1982, I took care of a man with serious heart disease. He had a previous history of a heart attack, ventricular arrhythmia and underwent coronary artery bypass surgery because of an unsatisfactory quality of life. He spent approximately three years under my care and in the latter two years I had close to 25 interactions with him; he was seen in the office, the emergency room and was admitted to the hospital on three separate occasions. I had a lot of feeling for this individual. I took care of him as if he were my brother. Unfortunately, he was one of those patients who was extremely anxious about his condition. And why shouldn't he be? Patients with cardiovascular disease have a persistent fear about the possibility of sudden death. Often, symptoms in the chest cause panic, and many patients believe that this is the end. I believe that this was the case with my patient. After several interactions and multiple office visits, my patient continued to be symptomatic despite the most sophisticated medical and surgical interventions. Then one day, he decided to take his own life. I was horrified and shocked over the loss of this man. I can remember speaking to his wife on the phone and feeling the depth of her despair and sorrow. I also wasn't prepared to lose a patient in this way. Nor was I prepared for the lawsuit that followed.

To be sued over a case like this was one of the most heartbreaking experiences I have ever had in my life. I was shamed, humiliated and felt betrayed. The fear of lawsuits is inherent in every physician and, unfortunately, it is becoming a sign of our times. Multiple depositions, telephone calls and attorney interactions finally culminated in a three-and-a-half week grueling trial. The legal process is a tedious, painstaking one. During the course of my trial, many things happened to my body over the threatened loss of a vital connection that was, in my case, self-esteem.

As a cardiologist and a psychotherapist, I knew perfectly well that the litigation drama could provide substrate for my own sudden cardiac death. I knew all too well and was familiar with the brain/heart hotline. I felt as if I were a criminal. After several depositions of "expert witnesses" who seemed to have no respect for the truth, I became frightened by the possibility of wearing the label of medical malpractice. I had difficulty sleeping for approximately five years. On the first day of the trial, I was put on the stand to be cross-examined by the prosecution. The cross-examination process went on for approximately three days. Although I was perfectly willing and open in telling my story, I felt that I could be tricked, trapped or seduced at any given moment. The plaintiff's attorney, in my mind, really had no respect for the truth; he wanted to win—at all costs.

As a doctor, I always considered myself battling the forces of nature, trying to keep people in harmony and out of disequilibrium with their bodies. I treated disease; I was a physician trying to heal and prevent illness. I had tremendous self-esteem, especially in emergency situations, but I wasn't prepared for legal battles. I was also a man with real heart and feeling and this encounter was heart wrenching, to say the least. I remember going to court and leaving many sick people behind in the hospital. I felt I was betraying my patients by being in court. But not defending myself would be a betrayal of the truth. Facing the shame of a plaintiff's verdict of being a "bad doctor" was overwhelming. I had many internalized emotions including anger, sadness, fear and vigilance. This stress caused my back to buckle, causing two bulging disks in my lumbosacral spine. At one point, I could not even walk and had to use a Tens walking unit to assist me in getting through the courtroom experience. A Tens unit uses vibrational energy to help soften the contracted tissues in the back.

The lawsuit was literally breaking my back. I felt as if I were at a Salem witchcraft trial when the plaintiff's witnesses twisted and distorted the evidence.

So many new feelings, once buried, came up for me during the trial. I felt so hurt that I cried. It was one of the first times that I had spontaneously cried since the days of my "ironman" training. In my education as a psychotherapist, I had spent many years learning that crying was beneficial to the heart; yet, I was never able to cry. I have always had difficulty with crying, which I saw reflected in many of my male patients who succumbed to heart disease. Therefore, I knew that I was at risk for a heart attack; crying was essential to release my heartbreak. Crying was also necessary to heal my heart.

In my anguish and dread, I had the feeling of hopelessness. I felt helpless and was at the mercy of others. Then I thought, "This is what it must be like for my patients who have succumbed to a heart attack. Hopeless!" My body was aching in this experience; my heart was literally broken. Then I remembered the old Chinese proverb, "There is opportunity in crisis." I never gave up hope and I had a strong faith in the truth. I tried to find something positive during this drama and found that this was an opportunity for me to get into my deep feelings of shame and humiliation, which I carried from childhood. I dreaded the possibility of losing the case, which would result in failure, loss of self-esteem, and thereby a loss of the vital connection of my work. After all, I was a highly trained specialist in the field of cardiology and the threat of being declared incompetent was too much to bear. My vigilance was overwhelming. But my belief in good conquering evil paid off. I was cleared of all charges, which reinforced the validity of my pursuing the truth and placing my whole heart into this ordeal.

I am sure that, like me, many physicians worry about their patients. Developing relationships with patients over a period of time creates a closeness. If they suddenly become ill and sometimes terminal, it is heartbreaking for the doctor. I usually know their families and over time I really feel their struggle and appreciate how painfully vulnerable they are. It's so sad. Worrying about the possibility of litigation and lawsuit is yet another added stress. I remember thinking that if I had lost this case, my "opportunity in crisis" would be to go to an underdeveloped country and become a "real doctor." I fantasized about going into the Peace Corps to treat illness and be a healer without any of the bureaucracy, threats or fears. I thought this would be a heart-healing experience.

It turned out that the lawsuit was exactly what I needed at this time in my life. It was something that helped me get in touch with my own sadness and my own feelings. It allowed me to cry. I remember my attorney sitting with me at lunch and asking if I was crying again. He really did not understand how important crying was for me. I believe he looked at me as being rather weak and timid; however, I welcomed the crying and the sadness that was finally being released from my body. My days as an athlete, a hardworking student, and an "iron man" really shut down many of my feelings. To be immersed in this lawsuit was to have my feelings back. Even to this day, I really have no animosity or negativity toward the family that sued me. There was a lot of opportunity for me in that crisis.

Following that threatened loss of self-esteem, my life went through a series of other losses. I soon became separated from my wife and we eventually divorced. I lost my favorite uncle as a result of lung cancer and then I had the heartbreaking experience of losing my father in my arms. Fortunately, experiencing deep feelings and the revitalization of old and new connections carried me through the heartbreak. I was able to work through my despair and feelings with much opportunity and hope. I was indeed fortunate. In others, however, sudden loss can provoke feelings of fear and panic which can lead to devastating consequences.

A recent example of such tragic loss occurred in the cardio-logical practice of one of my colleagues in Manchester, Connecticut. A 70-year-old man with a history of heart disease was outside raking his yard. He was suddenly stricken with a heart attack. Teenagers passing by found him lying near the front porch. The paramedics were summoned. His wife, a 72-year-old woman, was inside watching television, unaware of her husband's grave situation. As the paramedics were performing CPR, she ran over to her husband in a panic. Her last words before she collapsed were, "I can't live without him." She died suddenly. A postmortem showed they both had suffered heart attacks, but the wife actually had had a small heart attack two days prior to the sudden death of her husband. Thus, a previous small heart attack in combination with an unexpected, devastating loss provided the substrate for sudden cardiac death. Such a sudden loss provoked the brain with overwhelming feelings of panic and hopelessness leading to ventricular fibrillation in a heart that was already vulnerable. The wife died from the shock of seeing her moribund husband. There are multiple cases on record that mimic such events.

Dr. George Engel, an analyst and an internist, studied 275 cases of sudden cardiac death. A summary of his findings indicated that 20 percent of individuals dying from sudden heart attacks recently had experienced bad news about a loved one. Another 20 percent were experiencing acute grief at the time of their sudden death. Another 27 percent of individuals had a fear of personal injury or damage. In almost every case, some psychological stress occurred before the unexpected event of the sudden cardiac death. Briefly, some of Engel's cases included the following:

- A 40-year-old father was reported to slump dead as he cushioned the head of his son lying injured in the street beside his overturned motorcycle.

- A man, age 43, died suddenly after his 15-year-old son, faking a kidnap, called over the phone saying, "If you want to see your son alive, don't call the cops".

There are numerous cases in Engel's study that relate to sudden unexpected death occurring immediately after being told of the loss of a loved one.

In my own clinical practice, I too have experienced the sudden loss of patients. Being a critical care specialist, I have been able to interview "survivors" of the sudden death experience. Survivors successfully resuscitated were able to verbalize their feelings and their activities just prior to their sudden death experience. Let me share with you some case reports of sudden death.

CASE #1

Andy, a man in his late 40's, was admitted to our coronary care unit with an acute heart attack. On the evening of his admission, he was sleeping comfortably. He was dreaming. In his dream, he was walking with his father when he was a 12-year-old boy. Although Andy felt good about being with his father, he felt tremendous anguish when his father left him in the dream. Andy now started to panic as the dream reawakened his boyhood despair. When he was really 12, his father had left the family as a result of a messy divorce. The 12-year-old boy in the dream was experiencing deep sadness and longing over the loss of his father. Suddenly in the dream, my patient saw a white light shining through the forest. As he was then floating above the forest and saying goodbye to his father, he suddenly felt a crushing blow to his chest.

He awakened with several nurses frantically moving about his bedside. Fortunately, he was being monitored with an electrocardiogram at the time he was sleeping. He had suddenly experienced ventricular fibrillation and, with the swift decision of a nurse, he was brought back to life with a defibrillator. The dream revealed the estrangement from his father; the resulting intense longing brought up loss of hope. Reliving the experience as a 12-year-old boy in the dream recreated the loss of a vital connection. Although he experienced a near sudden death, he became a survivor with successful CPR. This case illustrates the all-too-common feelings of sadness and deep longing in the setting of a vulnerable heart.

CASE #2

The loss of job, self-esteem and purpose in living is reflected in Carl, a 60-year-old sports writer. Carl was an avid tennis player who was in terrific shape. Due to his "old age," he was forced to retire from the newspaper. He felt considerable resentment and anger toward his employers. Although he accepted his retirement with dignity and did not outwardly show anger, his dreams reflected the truth. His dreams were full of deep feelings of sadness and despair. In his dreams, he was reexperiencing the feelings of being needed. That is, his dreams consisted of his employers wanting him back on the job. Carl's job, in reality, gave him a purpose in living. The loss of his job for him was the loss of a vital connection. Since Carl could not find a new job, he had deep resentful feelings of anger and rage. The held-in explosive quality of these feelings resulted in an attack of ventricular arrhythmia leading to urgent hospitalization and treatment of his cardiac rhythm disorder.

The heartbreak of retirement may be seen in situations where sudden cardiac death actually becomes a maladaptive exit from a life without purpose or satisfaction. When your identity becomes your job, you become very vulnerable.

CASE #3

Jean was a woman in her early 60s who had been married for approximately 38 years. After discovering that her husband had become involved with another woman, she experienced deep feelings of anger, rage, humiliation and resentment. After four days of panic realizing that her husband was lost, she became crushed and gave herself permission to die. Jean stated, "After 38 years of marriage, how could I give up hope? I could never give up hope. However, after he bought a boat and planned to live on it with her, I finally accepted reality and experienced the loss. At first I was running around like a nut, driving myself crazy. I had the feeling that I had become a mad woman."

What really mattered to Jean was the hope; and with the loss of hope, she experienced a sense of doom. Panic surfaced; she developed sudden cardiac chest pain and collapsed. She was rushed to the emergency room by the paramedics and was found to be in ventricular fibrillation. She was successfully resuscitated. After several days of a stormy hospitalization, she required further evaluation including a cardiac catheterization which defined the anatomy of the blood vessels surrounding the heart. As we suspected, Jean had normal coronary arteries and did not experience a heart attack. Rather, she experienced acute heartbreak. Heartbreak was manifested by the cascade of a loss of hope, sense of doom, panic and ventricular fibrillation. Obviously, like voodoo death, this was a maladaptive escape. Sudden death was a way out. Once again, the feeling of intense loneliness, despair and rage can trigger a kind of suicide.

In contemporary society, an article in the *New England Journal of Medicine* concluded that survivors of myocardial infarction who became socially isolated or lonely died more often than the people who had supportive, nurturing environments. Thus, loneliness, like voodoo death, can really be a harbinger of a maladaptive escape. If one could adapt to the situation, one would not have the feeling of being trapped. But adaptability is a variable phenomenon. If we look at those suffering a bereavement, sudden death is two to ten times higher than in the general population. It is even worse if a man loses his wife than if a woman loses her husband. In general, women can adapt better than men. Women express feelings more often. Women find joy in sharing their deepest feelings, particularly with other women. Women form networks and nurture one another. Men, on the other hand, tend to build walls and hold feelings in. They keep secrets and will not communicate. Women are softer, less contracted and expand more easily than men. The feminine side has a "taking in" quality, whereas men are programmed to be harder, performance-oriented and do not have the instinctive ability to take in. They possess instead a learned ability to shut out. Women do a lot to release tension: They cry more easily, they menstruate (nature's way of releasing tension on a monthly basis) and they have the ability of total surrender of heart and body. A women's physiology is more in harmony and balance than a man's. Therefore women generally can emerge from crisis situations better than men. Women are really the stronger sex in regard to adaptability, flexibility, communication and establishing new vital connections after loss.

This maladaptability of males is illustrated in the following animal study that was performed on baboons in the Soviet Union. Baboons are very much like humans. They nurture one another. They also mate for life. The Russian investigators reared baboon couples and then took the male out of the cage and put a new male in. The ex-mate was placed only a few feet away in another cage in full view of his partner. This was a very cruel study to do to such sensitive animals. What the experiment showed was that all 18 of the male baboons, the "ex-husbands," died within six months of separation of stroke, hypertension and heart attack. Again, the acute psychological stress of being trapped, heartbroken and helpless overwhelmingly resulted in death.

Conversations of loss of hope can be the lethal messenger between the heart and the brain. There is growing evidence, for example, that chemical factors, influenced by central nervous system activity, can enhance cardiac arrhythmia and cause sudden cardiac death. Terrible disappointments have also been known to render individuals susceptible to sudden cardiac death. Such is the case in the story of the Andersonville prison.

History tells us that during the early stages of the Civil War, some prisoners were exchanged after months of containment and others were sent back once again to battle. But near the end of the war, Grant realized that the South was losing manpower. The idea of exchange was cancelled. The prison at Andersonville in southern Georgia was an area of approximately 15 acres that contained 30,000 federal prisoners of war. The conditions in this prison were intolerable to say the least. These men had very little food. There was no shelter and no drinking water. Many died of disease and exposure. They were overcrowded and, during the winter months, they had to walk through the night to avoid freezing to death. Stories concerning these prisoners were horrible. What kept these men going, however, was the hope in their hearts. This hope was sustained by rumors of exchange. Rumors of exchange were planted by Confederate spies infiltrating the Union ranks. The Confederate contingency feared the possible rebellion of 30,000 prisoners of war. They certainly did not have enough manpower to control such a rebellion. So the Confederate staff planted spies in the Union ranks to talk about plans to exchange. The prisoners were desperate. Rumors of exchange gave them the hope they needed to survive. If these rumors were believed, plans to escape were cancelled. Southern offi-

cers maintained these rumors to avoid mass turmoil or upris-
ing. In *The Soldier's Story*, author W. Goss, states,

> These two months were the most terrible of any experienced
> by the general prisoners. Nine thousand were said to have died
> during that space of time. In one day in August, no less than
> 160 prisoners died and the average was over 200 daily. From
> the first of February to the 16th of September, 12,000 Federal
> soldiers, prisoners of war, were carried from the prison to Dead
> Man's Trench and burial. Many of the deaths were hastened
> by despondency. After an unusual excitement about exchange,
> expecting to be called out and to be released at any moment,
> followed by disappointment, deaths were the most frequent.

This scenario clearly demonstrates the impact the loss of
hope had upon these soldiers' lives. In essence, this data supports W.A. Green's data of depression followed by acute psychological arousal providing the substrate for the sudden
death experience. What the author is describing is sudden cardiac death as a result of the loss of all hope, and sense of
doom. Panic, entrapment and death were the outcome. This
stimulation of the sympathetic nervous system against the
background of depression created a substrate for the sudden
death situation. Adaptability was not out of the question; yet
the only way out for some of these poor unfortunates was
death.

The Andersonville prisoners were imbued with the fear of
death. Fear is one of the most negative visceral emotions that
we experience. In voodoo death, unmitigated fear can cause an
overwhelming negative experience for the organism via overstimulation of the sympathetic nervous system rendering the
individuals susceptible to sudden cardiac death. To avoid fear
and terror, one would welcome death.

Fear can be a deadly emotion with dire consequences. For
example, after the Custer massacre, some of the Indian chiefs

testified that soldiers were shooting themselves in the head. There was an unwritten law among soldiers when fighting in hopeless situations: always save the last bullet for yourself. To be taken alive guaranteed a slow, painful death. In the Fetterman massacre a few years prior to Custer, the two highest ranking officers each had clean bullet wounds in their temples, indicating that each of them had shot himself during the hopeless battle. Acute fear can seduce the brain to self-destruct with self-inflicted wounds.

In our inquiry of sudden death, fear is an integral component. For example, Engel, who was an analyst, psychiatrist and internist, studied sudden death in painstaking detail. Was his study of sudden death a projection of something more? Perhaps he was afraid of his own death. In a conference several years ago, I heard Engel speak about his "nemesis" complex, which is when you believe that something tragic will happen to you. Like voodoo death, a nemesis complex is almost like placing a curse upon yourself. For example, Engel's father died of a myocardial infarction when Engel and his twin brother were young boys. It was very interesting to hear Engel eloquently speak about his own fear of dying from a fatal heart attack on the anniversary date of his father's death. While Engel did not fulfill the prophesy, his twin brother did. Engel did not die. Instead, he was admitted to the hospital with bleeding hemorrhoids. From an energetic point of view, Engel's bleeding hemorrhoids and subsequent anemia were a release of energy and tension that he was holding perhaps in his nemesis belief. It is similar to the release of energy in a menstruating woman, which frees up tension and contraction in the body. Engel's bleeding hemorrhoids probably saved his life and ended his obsession with the nemesis complex.

Many patients in my practice, particularly the young, have had an incredible nemesis—fear. They, like Engel, think that they will die of a heart attack because their father or mother died of a heart attack when they were young children. This fear of death is a major factor in many of the panic disorders that physicians treat. Treating panic disorders of this type is very delicate and requires the skill of a psychotherapist. Many of my patients who possess this complex are acutely in touch with the intense negativity and fear that goes on in their minds. Emotional healing in these individuals requires the virtual reprogramming of their belief systems. The danger in the nemesis complex is that the event which is so feared to happen may actually happen. People are powerful. People can create their own disease situations and therefore their own destiny. Fear in itself is a tremendously negative emotion that can deleteriously affect the heart. Like held-in, unreleased anger, fear requires a significant degree of aerobic and anaerobic energy. These negative passions are associated with increased levels of peripheral vascular resistance and increases in heart rate and cardiac output, which may create an undesirable burden on the cardiovascular system. The results of such fear can be seen on both the individual and societal levels.

If one looks at the various cultures in the world, one sees that the highest incidence of heart disease occurs in Finland. Now why would Finland have the highest incidence of heart disease in the world? It is true that some Finns smoke and that Finns eat a diet high in dairy and meat products. But the Swedes and the Norwegians also possess these habits and have a much lower rate of heart disease than the Finns. If one looks at the geography of Finland, however, one sees that it borders the Soviet Union. In fact, the Finnish towns that border the Soviet Union have the highest prevalence of coronary disease in the world. This occurs both in the young and old populations. What is it about the Finnish-Soviet border? Although I have never been there, I have been told by some of my colleagues that the border, even today, is one of barbed wire, tanks, guard dogs and artillery pointing at the Finnish people. Imagine what it would be like for a young child growing up in a town where devastation is only a few yards away. Could a young child mirror the fear of a parent? And if so, does fear become the prevailing risk factor that molds one's destiny? Both psychiatrists and psychotherapists agree that children do mirror the energies of their parents. Such mirroring can certainly affect the developmental process, and especially form and deform the circulatory system.

It is also interesting to note that the cultures with the most protective child rearing societies have the lowest incidence of heart disease. For example, in Japan, southern Yugoslavia, southern Italy and Greece, mothering and nurturing the child are cultural traditions; such loving protection and unconditional love are healthy for the heart. It is no wonder that heart disease is lowest in these cultures. Perhaps there is less fear, threat or vigilance in these families and more comfort, unity and togetherness.

Vigilance is an interesting word. Vigilance is what we experience before we experience fear. It is like being on guard. It is like waiting for something to happen. You could say that the Finns are very vigilant in that they are always wary of confronting the Soviets because of the previous unsuccessful war history. Vigilance will turn on hormonal pathways in the body that can have harmful effects upon the organism. For example, blood levels of potassium and HDL decrease while serum levels of cholesterol and adrenalin increase. We know that such hormonal imbalances can deleteriously effect the heart.

I remember when I was an intern at Albany Medical Center, I was the doctor for the professional wrestlers. Since I used to wrestle in high school and college, I took this job thinking that it would be interesting and a way to nurture my own interest in sports. What I did not realize was that the matches were all predetermined. It was kind of a show. Wrestlers acted, the referee acted and even the judges were acting. But what I also didn't realize was how frightened the wrestlers were. You see, a lot of the wrestlers were amateurs. They were not like real professionals; that is, they weren't fine-tuned machines who had exquisite control over their bodies. Although some of them had good control, many would lose control and consequently hurt their opponent. Sometimes they would make a. bad throw, or a fake punch might turn into a real punch. Although they were amateurs, they were all trying to make it in the professional ranks. When the crowds got crazy, the wrestlers would get crazy and a lot of them would get hurt. Sometimes they would dislocate shoulders, lose a tooth or even get a finger in the eye. They worried about breaking their necks and being paralyzed.

Before the wrestling started, "the doctor" was supposed to take their blood pressure. I was absolutely amazed. They had blood pressures as high as 240/170 at rest. I could not believe it! I was a young intern, only 25-years-old, and I just could not believe how high these blood pressures were. I remember going to one of the referees and telling him that a particular person could not wrestle. He looked at me as if I were crazy. What I didn't know then was that what these men really needed to do was to go out and discharge their bodies. They really needed to wrestle and breathe and flex their muscles. These men were vigilant; that is, they were exceedingly on guard for something negative to happen. It was an acute fight/flight response which, once enacted, discharged their visceral vascular readiness. The muscular action uncoupled their cardiovascular response and their blood pressure then came down. No one ever suffered a stroke by wrestling.

I learned a lot by watching those wrestlers. I learned the powerful bodily response of vigilance and what it can do to the cardiovascular system. I remember in my own experience as a college wrestler that I too had feelings of vigilance. While I very seldom had fears of being hurt on a body level, I did have a fear of losing. Losing connotates a sense of failure. This has been a core issue in my life. To lose at wrestling brings up the unconscious core feelings of failure, low self-esteem, feelings of worthlessness. Wrestling has always been an integral part of my life. My experience in wrestling undoubtedly helped me in many of the emergency situations I found myself in as a cardiologist. Frequently we would have to perform and achieve in a flicker of time. Emergency cardiology, with the insertion of pacemakers, cardiopulmonary resuscitation and the treatment of massive heart attacks sometimes requires the lightning speed of a well-trained, razor-sharp, athlete. The vigilance that I learned as a wrestler, I now employ daily in my cardiological practice.

Vigilance is anticipating the future which, in some cases, can be put to good use. For example, when crossing the street on a dark evening, one needs to be vigilant for approaching vehicles. By the same token, a cardiologist needs to be vigilant when caring for critically ill patients; anticipating complications can be lifesaving.

However, as a younger cardiologist, I recall being overly vigilant and fearful working in certain crisis situations with some patients. Because a patient may mirror the doctor's fear, this may have a negative consequence for the patient. I remember the only complication I ever had in the cardiac catheterization laboratory was in a woman who was "scared stiff." As I looked into her fearful eyes, I too became fearful. When she saw that I was fearful, she stopped breathing and subsequently developed a perforation of her ventricle. Fortunately, she survived without any lasting damage. Just as the Finns are overly vigilant, so was I in this particular case. Like the Finnish children mirroring their parent's fear, my patient saw my fear and reacted on a body level with a cardiac complication.

A good doctor knows when he or she sees fear in a patient and knows fear can have serious consequences. Cardiologists are well aware of the role that panic and fear place on the heart. For example, when doctors admit patients to the coronary care units, we frequently use drugs such as minor tranquilizers to alleviate fear. Morphine is frequently used in reducing the chest pain of myocardial infarction, not only for its pain-relieving activities, but also for its anxiety-lowering properties. Drugs that also interfere with adrenalin-like substances, i.e., beta blockers, are frequently utilized in situations where psychological arousal and excessive quantities of adrenaline are being released. Assuaging acute psychological arousal in a CCU setting is a major factor in the prevention of complex ventricular arrhythmias and complications in the post-heart-attack period. Although pharmacological agents are extremely useful, human touch should not be underestimated in enhancing comfort and reducing arousal.

In some life-threatening situations, human contact is probably the most powerful antidote. As a critical care specialist, being involved in an extraordinary amount of life/death situations, I am particularly struck by the impact of the supportive aspects of family. The positive emotion of human contact and love given to critically ill patients, in my opinion, has reversed overwhelming odds in many life-and-death situations. I have had the experience of seeing multiple life/death situations influenced by the presence of family. For example, I can remember calling in two brothers in the early morning hours to see their mother who was dying as a result of a massive heart attack. She was slipping away. She looked comfortable. She was willing to accept death without struggle and was literally giving up. Drugs were to no avail. At this time I summoned the brothers to come to the bedside. When they held her hand and talked to her through the early morning hours, she began to respond. When she saw the sun come up, she decided that she wanted to live. She eventually walked out of the hospital. I am convinced it was the timing of the sons' contact that was critical to this woman's situation.

The case of Frank involves the unfortunate fatal outcome of a 60-year-old male who lingered on a tether of life and death for approximately 20 hours. Even though he finally succumbed, he showed an incredible will to live because of his family.

Frank was admitted to our coronary care unit with crushing chest pain and shortness of breath. His pain lasted for several hours and he was not responding to the usual therapeutic drugs. This was in the days before thrombolytic therapy, which miraculously melts away the clot that inhibits blood flow to the heart. After various catheters were inserted into his body and into his heart, he continued to deteriorate in spite of all the sophisticated monitoring and multiple drugs we had on hand. With an arterial line in place, we were able to monitor his blood pressure on a beat-to-beat basis, and his blood pressure was gradually continuing to fall to the point where he was losing mental processes. Blood flow diminished and urinary flow decreased. His condition, known as cardiogenic shock, was the result of a large area of heart being damaged due to the occlusion of major coronary vessels.

However, Frank accepted this situation and he surrendered to me; that is, he participated with me in his care. He trusted me with all his being. I sensed his driven will to live. At one point during the course of his acute illness, his blood pressure continued to drop despite all medical maneuvers. At this point, I called in the family.

Five members of his family were actually waiting in the lobby. They were called to the bedside. His sons and daughters were told of his terminal situation. They came to the bedside and each placed their hands on his arms, his hands, and his legs. His eyes rolled back in his head, his forehead began to sweat and his breathing was only maintained by the ventilator. As each family member stroked an extremity, Frank took in their contact. When one of the members of the family began to pray out loud, his blood pressure began to recover. On the oscilloscope, his pressure increased into the 40s, 50s, 60s, and finally into the 70s. At this time, he was able to grasp a hand. He was developing overt cerebral function. He even opened his eyes. He felt life in his body again! It was an incredible, emotional episode. Two of the nurses began to cry as the family and I witnessed a miracle of an individual returning from sure death.

I was convinced that it was the power of love, serenity and human contact that gave Frank the strength and will to maintain his life-sustaining functions. I thought I was seeing a religious miracle. Unfortunately, 12 hours later, Frank had refractory ventricular arrhythmias and finally expired. Nevertheless, it was the contact with his family that rallied him even for a few hours.

This is one case that I will never forget. Was it a true mystical experience or was it simple touching that evoked such healing for a short time? The gift that I learned from Frank is one that I incorporate into my practice. I make it a point to sincerely touch and make gentle eye contact with every one of my patients who come through my office. Sometimes such simple contact and acknowledgement of their struggle, suffering and pain is all that is necessary in enhancing the getting-well process. I frequently offer my simple contact as a nonverbal communication. The energy in my touch is an embodiment of my spirit which comes from the heart. It is this nonverbal communication that in my mind is really the art of healing.

CHAPTER 5

———— ✧ ————

Physical and Emotional Risk Factors for Heart Disease

Through our inquiry into the causes of heart disease and sudden cardiac death, we have demonstrated the undeniable link between the brain and the heart. There is definitely a heart/brain "hotline." The identification of people at risk for sudden death depends not only on the hidden possibilities of heart disease, but also on the psychological and emotional status of the one afflicted. Unconscious thoughts and drives appear to be cardinal factors as the links between the forces in our personality and neuroregulatory centers that control heart function. I call these the hidden emotional risk factors for heart disease.

By now most people are quite familiar with the physical risk factors for coronary heart disease. This model has long been the standard that cardiologists use in predicting the likelihood of coronary heart disease as well as acute cardiac events such as sudden death.

Physical Risk Factors

Physical risk factors, or predisposing conditions that adversely affect one's health, include heredity, environment and lifestyle habits. Collectively, the well-known cardiovascular risk factors for cardiovascular disease include cigarette smoking, high blood pressure, elevated cholesterol and high blood sugar. These are the major cardiovascular risk factors that have been investigated in the large population studies. Other risk factors, such as obesity, stress, sedentary lifestyle and Type-A behavior have also been cited in recent studies.

Since the majority of this research has mostly been of a statistical nature, such risk factors are based on large population trends and cannot predict what will happen to one individual. For example, the Framingham Heart Study, begun several decades ago and still ongoing, is looking into lifestyle habits that focus on these major cardiovascular risk factors and their relation to heart disease. The Framingham Study evaluated the natural history of heart disease in a small New England town. Physical examinations were administered to all individuals who participated in the study and their lifestyle, habits and risk factors were analyzed. The Framingham Study showed that persons with no risk factors have only a 2 percent incidence of heart attack as compared to a 47 percent incidence for those having five or more risk factors. Risk factors can be either controllable or uncontrollable. The controllable risk factors include cigarette smoking, high blood cholesterol, high blood pressure, obesity, diabetes, Type-A personalities, stress and sedentary lifestyle. The uncontrollable risk factors include being male, increasing age and having a family history of heart disease.

Uncontrollable Risk Factors

HEREDITY, AGE AND GENDER

Although coronary heart disease increases with advancing age, heart attacks are still very prevalent under the age of 40. Although generally men are more often afflicted than women, the incidence of heart attacks has been increasing in women, especially within the last two decades.

WOMEN AND HEART DISEASE

I worry about the fact that so many women still think heart disease is primarily a problem for men. The truth is that heart disease is a major health risk for women, but many physicians did not realize this until recently, so they've done very little to encourage their women patients to take steps to protect their health.

I am also concerned because much of our knowledge regarding heart disease has come from large clinical studies done on men. This leads many physicians to diagnose and treat women as if heart disease affected them the same way. Nothing could be further from the truth. Heart disease affects men and women very differently.

For instance, an American woman is five times more likely to develop heart disease than breast cancer. About 240,000 American women will die annually from coronary artery disease, compared with 50,000 who die from breast cancer. Cardiovascular disease such as stroke and heart attack kills more women annually than any other illness including all the cancers combined. Despite this, recent surveys still indicate that misdiagnosis, underdiagnosis and lack of effective treatment for heart disease are still very common for women today.

Since most cardiologists still see heart disease as a male phenomenon, they treat women less effectively and less aggressively than they treat men, often with catastrophic results.

For example, if a 45-year-old woman and a 45-year-old man both come to the emergency room with chest pain, most physicians will probably admit the man and tell the woman that her symptoms are due to stress and anxiety. This is because most doctors are trained to believe that cardiovascular disease has a low probability in women. Not many realize that among peri- and postmenopausal women, the incidence of coronary events quadruples as women approach middle age (45 years old and older). Unfortunately, I see more and more cases of coronary heart disease in postmenopausal women.

Statistically, the outlook for women who suffer a myocardial infarction is more grim than for men. They have a poorer prognosis. Studies indicate increased mortality, both during hospitalization and at one year postdischarge. Women also have a higher mortality rate with angioplasty and coronary artery bypass surgery. Following surgery, they have more complications and a more difficult psychological adjustment.

In addition to advancing age and gender, family history is yet another uncontrollable risk factor. Some cardiologists believe that family history is a major consideration, but others, myself included, feel that family history is significant only if the child mirrors or models parental actions, behaviors or habits. The term "psychological genetics" is becoming more and more popular among cardiologists. For example, if a parent died of a heart attack at age 40 and if the child models the parent's behavior in terms of smoking, diet, sedentary lifestyle, personality, etc., the child is indeed at great risk for heart attack. On the other hand, if a child models the other parent who has, perhaps, a much more favorable risk profile, the incidence of heart disease is less likely. Although genetics play an important role in diseases such as diabetes, high blood pressure and hereditary hypercholesterolemia, in terms of the global cardiac risk factor model, family history has less influence when the habits and lifestyle characteristics of a child are different than the parental cardiac victim. Thus, a positive family history of heart attack does not necessarily mean that one is doomed by his or her genes. Rather, it is a gift that warns one to pay special attention to the controllable risk factors. By reducing the controllable risk factors, it is possible to minimize the cardiovascular risk. This is a crucial point in preventive medicine.

Controllable Risk Factors

CIGARETTE SMOKING

The relationship of cigarette smoking to heart disease has been extensively studied and is now generally accepted. People who smoke 20 or more cigarettes a day are more likely to suffer a heart attack than those who smoke less than 10 or none at all. The basis for the harmful effects of cigarette smoking upon the heart may be the effect of nicotine upon the arteries. Nicotine has a constrictive effect upon the arteries and presumably also upon the coronary arteries.

Nicotine can also cause blood platelets to stick together, thereby enhancing the vulnerability to coronary thrombosis. Since a heart attack is due to constriction with thrombosis of one of these arteries cutting off the blood supply to the heart muscle, it is clear why the Surgeon General's warning against smoking was justified. Smoking causes a buildup of carbon dioxide and carbon monoxide that not only damages the small blood vessels, but also takes oxygen away from the heart. Recent investigations have revealed a greater incidence of silent myocardial ischemia in smokers, as the buildup of nicotine and carbon monoxide distorts one's perception of pain by increasing the pain threshold. Thus, smoking is extremely hazardous not only in provoking and initiating symptoms by its direct toxic effects, but it also results in reduced sensations, thereby delaying any early warning of distress. Statistically speaking, smokers are almost twice as likely to have a heart attack as nonsmokers. Smokers also experience more sudden cardiac death.

DIET

Another area of intensive investigation in the search for causative factors in heart disease is the diet. For one thing, the atheromatous plaque that develops in the arteries is part of the disease known as atherosclerosis. Hardening of the arteries, as atherosclerosis is commonly called, is formed by the deposit of cholesterol and saturated fatty acids in the artery walls.

Because the liver produces all the cholesterol the body needs, a diet high in saturated fat (the building blocks for cholesterol) can flood the vascular system, thereby contributing to the development of atherosclerosis. Cholesterol is a waxy substance derived from the diet or manufactured by the body from ingested fats. The body uses cholesterol to build cells, manufacture bile salts and sex hormones. Cholesterol cannot be dissolved in liquids because fats are insoluble in water. Since blood is mostly made up of "sea water," cholesterol cannot be dissolved in the bloodstream and needs a carrier for transport. Two types of carriers that transport cholesterol are LDL and HDL.

Low-density lipoprotein (LDL) is the "bad" kind of carrier, which deposits cholesterol in the lining of the arteries. Too much LDL leads to the development of fatty deposits in the vascular system. A large number of studies have shown that high levels of LDL cholesterol are associated with an increased risk of heart attack. Lowering these levels reduces the risk. Levels greater than 160 mg/deciliter are considered high and deleterious to your health. Levels below 130 mg/deciliter are considered desirable. It is important to remember that LDL levels can be lowered by decreasing your intake of saturated fat; thus eating a prudent lowfat diet is a major factor in lowering LDL.

High-density lipoprotein (HDL) is the "good" kind of carrier. HDL picks up excess cholesterol and delivers it to the liver for further processing. Since HDL is important in carrying cholesterol away from the artery walls, the higher the level, the greater the protection from coronary artery disease. Levels of HDL less than 25 are considered very dangerous and levels greater than 60 are very protective for the heart. HDL levels can be increased by regular exercise, by not smoking and by maintaining an ideal body weight.

A profound connection between diet and cardiovascular disease becomes evident when disease statistics from various cultures clearly show that increasing one's cholesterol increases the chances of developing heart disease.

The typical American diet is overloaded with deadly quantities of highly saturated fatty foods that overwhelm the vascular system. Thus, it is not surprising that Americans have a much higher incidence of heart disease than the Japanese or Mediterranean population, who tend to take in very little fat and whose diets are low in animal and dairy products. In the culture of the African Bantu, whose diet is mostly beans, grains vegetables and fruit the average total cholesterol level is approximately 90-100 mg/dl, and coronary heart disease is a rare occurrence.

Recent research indicates that the Japanese and Mediterranean diets offer far less risk for cardiovascular disease. This is due not only to the reduced fat intake, but also because these vegetable-rich diets contain abundant levels of phytonutrients such as carotenoids and flavonoids that protect one from developing coronary heart disease.

Phytonutrients are natural disease fighters which plants have developed over the years to protect them against disease as well as insects. Research has shown that phytonutrients yield similar benefits to the people who eat them. There are many different types such as flavonoids, carotenoids, polyphenols, turpenoids, ligans, carbinols, indoles and sulphorophanes, to name a few. Studies on phytonutrients have shown that people in various cultures who eat more fresh fruits and vegetables have a lower incidence of heart disease and cancer. Consider the fact that the Northern European populations of Scotland and Scandinavia have a far greater incidence of coronary heart disease than do the Southern Mediterranean countries of Greece, Italy and Yugoslavia. American men between the ages of 55 and 59 experience coronary heart disease death nearly eight times more often than Greek men of the same age. Diets rich in phytonutrients are especially valuable in preventing heart disease because they not only lower cholesterol, but prevent the oxidation of cholesterol into an atherosclerotic plaque. The Japanese and Mediterranean diets are also rich in antioxidants and favorable fats such as monounsaturated olive oil in the Mediterranean diet and the linolenic acid of soy products in the Japanese diet. The Mediterranean diet also features red wine which can also prevent the oxidation of LDL

Similarly, the Japanese drink considerable quantities of green tea which not only can lower cholesterol levels but can prevent oxidation as well. Both of these diets also contain large quantities of fiber-rich legumes and grains which also help prevent LDL buildup. Both diets also feature abundant amounts of garlic and other health-enhancing herbs that have been used as cures since antiquity.

Thus, whether negatively or positively, cholesterol, phytonutrients, fiber and saturated fatty acids are implicated in the clogging action of atherosclerosis. Since most afflicted individuals have above-normal levels of cholesterol and lipids in their blood, reducing their dietary intake of these substances makes good sense. This hypothesis was tested in a research project that led to the conclusion that restricting the intake of animal fats does have some effect on the development of heart disease. This study, like the one dealing with smoking, is a statistical analysis of probability. While it does indicate that there is some connection between diet and heart disease, it does not prove that heart disease is directly due to an improper diet alone. Although diet is a major factor, it is not the only one. However, all cardiologists need to counsel their patients about diet therapy, cholesterol lowering and the health benefits of antioxidants and phytonutrients. For a more in-depth analysis of diet, nutritionals and heart disease, see my recent book, *Optimum Health: A Lifesaving Prescription for Your Body and Mind.*

HYPERTENSION

High blood pressure in multiple clinical research studies has been shown to be a significant risk factor in cardiovascular disease. The incidence of stroke, congestive heart failure, and diseases of the aorta are all increased as one's blood pressure rises. Everyone's blood pressure varies during the course of a day. For example, it may be lower during episodes of quiet or restful activity, particularly during sleep. Blood pressure may suddenly rise during times of activity, exercise, stress and, particularly, held-in emotional feeling. Blood pressure is generally lower in the younger age groups and rises with advancing age. Although there is some disagreement over what is too high and what is too low, cardiologists in general agree that the lower the numbers, the better it is for the patient. High blood pressure is considered to be suspect if the systolic pressure is greater than 140 and the diastolic reading is more than 90 mm of Mercury.

There are usually no symptoms with hypertension. High blood pressure causes an augmented force in blood vessels, thereby weakening the cellular walls and allowing for increased deposition of noxious bodily and environmental toxins. Such toxins as nicotine and harmful cholesterol deposits (LDL) may infiltrate the walls of these damaged vessels, thereby allowing the proliferation of plaque buildup. As the plaque builds up, blood platelets may stick to the walls, thereby causing the coronary thrombosis resulting in a myocardial infarction. Although high blood pressure alone is a serious risk factor, in combination with other risk factors it increases one's chances of having a myocardial event exponentially. Maintaining a normal blood pressure, therefore, is essential for one's health.

Approximately 10 percent of hypertension is caused by some structural or metabolic abnormality in the body. Ninety percent of hypertension, however, is related to a multitude of factors. Some individuals at birth may have genetic weaknesses and may be predisposed to develop hypertension. Others are prone to environmental stress and the perils of increased salt intake. This was clearly identified in some of the cultures of the Caribbean. Natives who cooked their food in sea water seemed to develop increased high blood pressure, whereas those who cooked with tap water had less incidence. Blood pressure can usually be lowered by the use of targeted nutritional supplementation supported by pharmacological agents, reduced salt intake, reduction of stress and particularly by weight loss in people who are overweight.

OBESITY

Being overweight endangers the heart in several ways. It is a major contributor to heart disease. By itself, it also has a metabolic relationship to higher cholesterol and blood sugar levels. For example, overweight people are much more likely to develop diabetes in the adult years.

Obesity, even if only mild to moderate, increases the risk of coronary heart disease, especially for middle-aged women. This was recently seen in a large population study involving 115,886 women which concluded that being overweight is a major cause of morbidity and mortality from coronary heart disease. Although obesity also affects the other risk factors of hypertension, high cholesterol and high blood sugar, the pattern of body fat distribution also has important ramifications. For example, fat concentrated in the abdomen and upper body appears to be more strongly associated with hypertension, high blood sugar and abnormal levels of serum cholesterol than fat concentrated in the lower body and hips. Thus, maintaining good body weight not only affects one's outside appearance, but also has profound physiological structural effects that can eventually lead to serious heart disease in addition to diabetes.

BLOOD SUGAR

Another common risk factor for cardiological disease is high blood sugar or diabetes. The Framingham data indicated that whatever the risk-factor profile, high blood sugar doubles the risk. Diabetes, a condition which contributes to hardening and narrowing of the arteries, is a gradual degenerative process that contributes to heart disease. Obesity, increased fat in the blood, and high blood pressure are frequently seen in individuals predisposed to a diabetic condition. Once again, maintaining a normal body weight and utilizing a prudent diet low in sugar and fat content may help delay or prevent the damaging effects of high blood sugar. Regular exercise is also extremely important.

SEDENTARY LIFESTYLE

Sedentary lifestyle is also considered an important risk for coronary heart disease. Population studies, for example, have suggested that increased physical activity has a favorable impact on cardiac events. This was clearly seen in a study of 500 sedentary bus drivers in England who were compared with the more active bus conductors. On autopsy it was found that there was a much higher incidence of coronary heart disease among the drivers who sat all day as opposed to the bus conductors who walked up and down the stairs of the double-decker English buses. In a study of San Francisco longshoremen, active physical labor also seemed to be a major factor in reducing the incidence of heart disease. A study of Harvard alumni with a long-term follow-up of at least 15 years showed that those who regularly exercised and expended approximately 2000 calories per week (the equivalent of walking seven miles per week) had a lower annual mortality rate than those who did not participate in regular physical activity.

The impact of physical exercise was also intuitively known by primitive man. He knew that through ritual dances his body would gain strength for future physical and psychological stresses. Among the ancient Spartans, to be physically inactive was considered to be a discredit to one's honor and character. In more modern society, Hans Selye advised that man should not avoid work, but should find the work that best suits him for successful activity even in advancing age. People who exercise regularly tend to have a lower blood pressure, a more ideal body weight and a better balance of HDL and LDL cholesterol. Exercise has multiple biochemical, structural and psychological benefits. A detailed description of exercise, including energy-releasing bioenergetic exercises, will be discussed in a later chapter.

Emotional Risk Factors

The second major category of risk factors includes the psychological or behavioral factors that cause chronic or immediate stress in the individual. Psychological risk factors are related to personality type, experience and adaptability, as well as to behavioral and cultural factors. This may explain why one individual responds to a stressful event by developing disease while another does not. For example, maladaptive coping mechanisms such as smoking, overeating, overuse of alcohol and hypertension, are frequently seen as an individual's response to chronic stress.

The psychological risk factors can be just as lethal as the more accepted physical risk factors. Although the epidemiological relationship between physical risk factors and heart disease is important to consider, it is also essential to note that the major physical risk factors (cigarette smoking, increased cholesterol, hypertension) are found in less than half of those who succumb to coronary artery disease. Therefore other factors must be considered. It is my belief that hidden emotional risk factors are the missing link. I believe that heart health depends on paying attention to the profound physical effects that emotions have upon the body. Emotions express themselves as behaviors and as physiological reactions that can place one at risk for heart disease. These are the "hidden risk factors" in heart disease which many cardiologists fail to acknowledge.

Since it is agreed that chronic psychosocial stress can lead to unhealthy behaviors such as excessive smoking and inappropriate diet, it is clear that modern man's personality and reactivity to stress are key ingredients in heart disease. There is also strong evidence that suggests a connection between psychological conflict, excessive and prolonged arousal and the etiology of coronary heart disease or systemic hypertension. Other important biobehavioral interactions such as Type A behavior and hostility also appear to be linked to coronary heart disease. Thus, when we discuss cause and relationship in heart disease, we have to consider not only the physical risk-factor relationships, but also the biobehavioral or emotional components. We need to think of traditional risk factors as an extension of our personality traits. Even though anger, hostility and rage are legitimate components of our personalities, most of us are hesitant to acknowledge this "shadow" or "dark side" of ourselves. As a result, we often deny or suppress these feelings and are not even aware of them. But I think that getting in touch with these powerful hidden emotions and becoming aware of their contribution to heart disease is critical to healing and protecting the heart.

Consider high blood pressure. Although it may be caused by a chemical imbalance, unhealthy diet or by being overweight, its alternative name, hypertension, gives a clue to another major cause. Could hypertension arise because someone is "hyper-tense," filled with bottled-up anger or rage? We have known for a long time that repressed anger is the most powerful "hidden" cause which contributes to high blood pressure. My work has convinced me that anger works the same way as a major cause of heart disease. We shall investigate anger in a subsequent analysis of the "dark side." It is important to understand behavioral and biological relationships. The mind/body connection can be either supportive or destructive. Again consider cholesterol.

Researchers have found an interesting connection between increased stress and blood cholesterol levels. Cholesterol can be grossly elevated by stress. It has been shown that such levels increase significantly at times of stress and time pressure regardless of the diet. This has been seen in accountants during tax season. Certified public accountants who were followed from January 1 to April 15 have demonstrated as much as a 100 mg/dl rise in serum cholesterol without a change in diet. Under such stressful conditions, cholesterol can be generated from the liver. Such was the case in my own personal study. Approximately 10 years ago I was asked to submit a fasting serum cholesterol for an insurance evaluation. Since I was performing three cardiac catheterizations that day, I asked that blood be drawn prior to 7:30 in the morning.

At that time, my blood cholesterol was 180 mg/dl. After performing two routine cardiac catheterizations, I had a third most stressing case of an individual with complex congenital heart disease. The cardiac catheterization was complicated by a cardiac arrest. The patient actually stopped breathing but was successfully resuscitated. The procedure took approximately five hours, requiring multiple catheters and multiple pharmacological interactions. I really sweated during this case. When the procedure was over, it was approximately three o'clock in the afternoon. I had had nothing to eat all day. As I was walking to the cafeteria, I passed the blood lab where

I had blood drawn earlier that morning. Since I had a strong belief in psychological stress and how it affects the body, I asked for a second blood test to be drawn. I was astonished to see the results. My blood cholesterol had risen to 240 mg/dl. Obviously my body reacted to the stressful events of the day, producing cholesterol in excessive amounts despite a fast of almost 20 hours.

A similar finding was seen in a study of medical students whose cholesterol levels were significantly elevated after being told that they had failed exams. Thus, we see that fear and vigilance raises our cholesterol. Conversely, loving contact lowers cholesterol. A study of rabbits that were cuddled and petted by animal handlers showed a lower rate of arteriosclerotic aortic lesions than did a mass group of controls that did not receive preferential care. This cuddling and simple contact confers a "protective effect" on the vascular system.

Humans are no exception. As trite as it may sound, love indeed heals. In my "Healing the Heart" workshops, we see profound cholesterol lowering when a patient experiences contact and connectedness in a supportive environment. In these four-to seven-day workshops, cholesterol levels have been lower in every one of our participants, with some losing as much as 100 mg/dl of cholesterol in just a few days! Although these participants were also eating a low-fat, high-fiber diet, the dramatic reduction in cholesterol supports the notion that emotional contact can positively affect our health.

Over time, holding in your emotions can make your blood more susceptible to cholesterol elevation. Although digging into your emotions and allowing yourself to be vulnerable can be difficult if you are unaccustomed to such soul-searching, I invite each of you to consider looking more deeply into your emotional self. Such introspection can initially be painful, but it is well worth the effort in the long run. When you support and nurture yourself, your more positive self-esteem reflects itself in healing the body. Such nurturing and protective influences on health were validated in other studies as well. In an animal model, a group of monkeys were fed the prudent diet recommended by the American Heart Association but were placed in an unstable living environment. Results showed that these monkeys had an excess of coronary heart disease as compared to the monkeys living in stable groups and fed the same diet.

This highlights the importance of social stress and behavioral demands as a crucial factor in a disease model regardless of the diet. It is also supported by another animal study which demonstrated that adrenalin injected into mammals, equal to amounts produced by emotional stress, elevated blood cholesterols.

When acute stresses are applied to humans, massive elevation in adrenalin occurs as well as increases in free fatty acids and triglycerides. This was seen in a study of race car drivers in England. High elevations in cholesterol and blood lipids occurred regardless of the diet. These drivers risked their lives in this endeavor, showing that this kind of physical risk-taking raises one's cholesterol and therefore heightens the risk of heart disease. Could the fear of death cause coronary disease? Consider the fact that American soldiers killed in the Korean War showed advanced atherosclerosis even among those who were only 19 years old. What caused the buildup of plaque? Was it smoking, diet, the stress of combat or were there other factors? It was not surprising to learn that several deaths in the Persian Gulf conflict were not attributed to combat wounds, but rather to acute heart attack. The fear of death is obviously a major psychological stress. Although one-half of all Americans will eventually develop some form of atherosclerosis, the prevalence of heart disease in such young men raises some intriguing speculations.

Even more puzzling is the fact that Chinese soldiers killed in action in Korea had far less coronary heart disease on autopsy analysis. Could culture and race render protection to the heart? As I mentioned earlier, less coronary heart disease also occurs in Southern European countries. In 1986 I had the opportunity to lecture in Belgium at an International Conference on Bioenergetic Analysis about the cultural aspects of heart disease. After considerable research on the topic, I came upon a paper which was extremely provocative.

During the course of 10 years, the heart attack rate of various European countries was recorded to see which countries had a higher incidence of heart disease. In the course of this study, it was astonishing to note that the Island of Crete did not report even one heart attack over a 10-year period as a cause of death in any of its inhabitants. At first I thought that the author of this study must have made a mistake. He stated that even though the cholesterol level was over 200 in the average inhabitant, the sunny climate and lack of stress must have been major positive factors in preventing heart attack. Today, we know that the Mediterranean diet, rich in monounsaturated fat such as olive oil and other antioxidants, has proved to be crucial in cardiovascular protection. But, the fact remains that the incidence of heart attack on this island was zero over a 10-year period. Therefore, some other factors must be taking an active role.

After I gave this lecture to an audience of approximately 300 participants, a question-and-answer period followed. During this time, a physician from Greece explained that the reason for the lack of heart disease in Crete and Greece was related to the healing powers of nurturing relationships, particularly among males. This doctor indicated that men in Crete spend quality time with one another. Over lunch they talk about real feelings. Money, sports and business—the favorite topics of American men—are not discussed. Rather, men talk about their feelings, their families, their dreams and even their spiritual beliefs. Also they do not wear a social mask. They argue, they cry, they support and they hold each other. This physician felt that such comradery, occurring often over games of chess and during a two-hour lunch, is a major factor in the reduction of coronary heart disease. As a psychotherapist, I completely agree with his hypothesis.

Although other cultural studies have emphasized physical

risk factors, such as the American Framingham Study, the impact of psychological and emotional risk factors on heart disease is much more recognized in other cultures. In 1987, Peter Nixon, a cardiologist in England with an international reputation on burnout and fatigue in heart disease asked me to write about my work on psychotherapy and heart disease for a British journal. Nixon, in contrast to many American cardiologists, had a strong belief in the importance of instructing his patients about how to heal themselves through rest and sleep.

It is so important for a patient to know that he or she can prevent and even heal heart disease through lifestyle choices of diet, exercise or even the use of nutritional supplements. However, many hidden risk factors also contribute strongly to heart disease. These are the powerful emotional and psychological causes of heart disease. They include suppressed anger, rage, the loss of love (what I call heartbreak) and the emotional isolation of the lack of intimacy with other people. Not having connections or the loss of a vital connection are crucial factors as well. These risk factors contribute to the development of heart disease as surely as smoking, a high-fat diet, stress, high blood pressure and lack of exercise. You can reduce the effects of these psychological risks by learning how to open your heart to your feelings, how to relax and minimize stress, how to breathe and how to build strong emotional connections with other people.

Based on my two decades of experience as a cardiologist and psychotherapist, I strongly believe that prevention is easier than cure when it comes to heart disease. I also believe that if you do have heart disease, you can slow its progression and even reverse it. In the next chapter, I will discuss the "shadow" and how its powerful forces can be integrated into healing the physical and emotional sides of your personality.

CHAPTER 6

───── ✍ ─────

The Shadow: Our Dark Side

Serious or even life-threatening illness can indeed be cata-strophic. It is a major, often prolonged, life-interrupting event accompanied by pain, anxiety and despair, plus a deep longing for things to be restored to normal. Unfortunately, in our society, "normal" is frequently not healthy and it may have been our "normal" patterns of feeling, thought and behavior that have brought us to this physical crisis point. Let me ex-plain how it happens.

We are all born with a natural capacity to release emotions as soon as they arise. If you have forgotten this, watch any baby to see how it is done. A baby is soft, fluid and at times out of control and demanding. The utterance of a cry is fre-quently the only way a baby can communicate. If you watch a baby who is upset, you see that the baby will cry or scream and that when he/she is finished, his/her body softens and he/she is peaceful and smiling again. When a baby is being nursed and held, he/she may also try to communicate with the mother by twisting and turning or even biting the breast. In essence, a baby's way of communicating is genuine, honest and very primitive.

If a mother responds to her baby's cries by ignoring them or even screaming back at the baby or shaking him, the infant over time will shut down emotionally. If reaching out to the outside world (mother) proves to be threatening, dangerous or frustrating the infant will often withdraw and stop expressing his or her needs in order to survive. The baby prefers to be safe.

Young growing children face a similar situation. We have all heard the familiar phrases "Don't cry or I will give you something to cry about," "Big boys don't cry," or "It's silly to be afraid." Unfortunately most parents give children many confusing messages about a very natural, human aspect of their being—their emotions. They are told to stop crying when they are hurt and need to cry, they are taught that crying is weakness, anger is not ladylike and that men should not be afraid. They are urged to "cheer up" when they feel sad. Many children have been treated disrespectfully and even abusively (physically or emotionally) through the years and have come to view this treatment as normal and to be expected. Some children are even hit, reprimanded or abandoned when they express certain emotions such as anger, sadness or fear.

The impact of all this repression is profound and tragic. After years and years of learned repression, of developing defense systems to disconnect and to not experience one's feelings, we have lost ourselves. We then wonder why we feel so alone, so separate and disconnected from ourselves and others. The ultimate separation is separation from yourself, from your feelings, from your needs, from your passion.

Where does all this emotional energy go? It becomes an unknown, painful, unresolved memory in our unconscious. From there, it descends into a deep place called the "shadow." The energy actually gets stuck in the body, in the muscles and in the cells. This unreleased energy becomes the seeds of *dis-ease*, of disharmony inside us.

Consider that generalized body tension can frequently be a manifestation of fear. If fear is repressed or denied as a reality, the body will compensate by exhibiting a specific attitude or tension. Most men who are afraid of their feelings of fear cover them up by an exaggerated expression of courage which is manifested in their body and attitude. Their shoulders may be squared off and raised, their chest inflated and abdomen sucked in. They are not really aware that their attitude is really a defense against fear until they find that they cannot drop their shoulders, relax their chest and breathing or let their abdomen relax. When such muscular tensions are released, fear is often then raised to consciousness.

However, if our intuition, growth and insight are stifled, some of our issues of unrecognized fear, anger and sadness are unconsciously acted out through feelings of hostility, cynicism, judgmentalism, self-imposed martyrdom or addictive behaviors of every description including codependency. It is, therefore, crucial that any comprehensive healing program include plenty of time to investigate the mysterious and convoluted landscape of the shadow where so much of our vital energy becomes trapped in early life. This was the case in my own personal therapy with John Pierrakos. Dr. Pierrakos feels that in order to evolve into higher spiritual growth, it is imperative to dig deep into the depths of our dark side.

For more than a year, I worked on the ugliest side of my personality. In my therapy with Alexander Lowen, as well as with other therapists, I unconsciously moved away from this side of my character. I really did not want to get in touch with it or even consider that I had these ugly emotions. Most of us, in general, do not want to admit that we have feelings of cynicism, rage, anger or hostility.

Much of the work I did with Dr. Pierrakos was feeling and experiencing the "monster" within. The therapy, at times, was incredibly powerful. The affective side of the work was the most profound I have ever done in psychotherapy. Pierrakos would ask me to focus on the ugly raging monster inside me. At times the verbal and hitting exercises were exhausting.

Following these intense therapeutic maneuvers, my body would soften and I would feel a gentle streaming of vibrations through my arms, legs and even my neck and thorax. After doing such profound and deep work, I found myself connecting more with my heart. For example, I told Pierrakos this story of when I was traveling in a train.

The Long Island Railroad has seats usually all facing in one direction; however, in some cars some of the seats allow the passengers to face each other. I was sitting in one such seat. One afternoon, after a session with Pierrakos, I was watching the rituals of many of my fellow passengers. Some were eating lunch, reading books and newspapers, others were putting on makeup and still others were sleeping. As the train was jerking and bobbing and as I was observing these people, I felt tremendous tranquility and love from deep within myself.

I felt a connection with everybody in the train car. As I felt my heart open, I began to experience feelings of love. It was truly a mystical experience I shall never forget. What caused such an experience? I am sure it had to do with the deep exploration of my dark side. As a cardiologist and psychotherapist, I can absolutely attest to the crucial value the shadow offers as a means of opening the chest and heart to love. But what actually is the "shadow?" And, can we really define it?

Defining the "Shadow"

When I speak of the shadow, I am referring to that part of the human psyche that provides a repository or a hiding place for our unacceptable impulses, desires, thoughts, feelings and emotions. It provides containment and safe storage for our hard-to-control energies and psychoemotional toxic waste, in the quiet holding chaos of the unconscious—those things which are too painful, too powerful or too threatening to face directly.

Yet, even the most horrific aspects of our personalities exist for a reason. The reason is really quite simple. There is a certain beauty in a mechanism such as this. It preserves and protects the child at the ego level, the level of the small self. This is especially important in childhood, when psychological survival is precarious and the child's resources are not yet under his or her control. Even our physical well-being is dependent upon the good intentions or the goodwill of another. The trouble arises when expectations formed during childhood interactions create filters through which we as adults unknowingly experience and interact with the world in a dysfunctional fashion.

A filter is a psychological construct. It is similar to a prism. We all know that a prism bends and twists light as it enters it. Similarly, if one bends and twists the incoming information, a distortion of reality will be created. When our beliefs become our perceptual filters, our experience of life cannot help but conform to whatever fits our preconceived construct of reality. Thus, our beliefs can mold our attitude about life. What began as self-protection and preservation will eventually create a distorted world view. Over time, this distorted perception leads to self-destructive patterns of adult behavior; unconscious reactions increasingly edge out or displace appropriate and thoughtful adult action. Somehow, we manage to remain blissfully unaware of what has happened below the level of our unconscious. Our singular world view becomes "the way things are" and our maladaptive strategies and behavior become "the way things are done here." We seek out relationships with those who share our own views and beliefs and come into conflict, often violent, with those who do not share our framework or paradigm. So we continue to generate circumstances and events that reaffirm these widespread, largely unconscious distorted patterns of belief and interaction. We view them as entirely "normal," but they are neither health-promoting nor life-enhancing when carried throughout adulthood.

We have already mentioned how the shadow functions to contain what we neither want to own or get in touch with. If we began to acknowledge the bad and ugly parts of ourselves, we must begin with the question: Who or what is inhabiting this subterranean holding tank in our unconscious?

The answers: Our dragons live there—guardians of a treasure. The dragons have names such as envy, jealousy, hatred, greed, lust, rage, fear and (one of the biggest dragons) the will to power, also known as the need to be in control. Even guilt, that furtive, self-effacing little beast, is a strategy for making ourselves wrong before someone else beats us to it. But let's not forget some of our favorite dragons—vanity, pride, arrogance and the need for self-aggrandizement. Even our suffering and our flaws are magnified and distorted when viewed through the shadow's looking glass. Thus we may become martyrs in our daily melodramas.

Was anyone ever so misunderstood, unappreciated, let down and taken for granted as we? Some day, "they" will know and appreciate all we really do for "them" (whoever they are). But by then, of course, it will probably be too late. Or what about the scenario that I frequently see among my coronary-prone patients. It goes something like this, "I know my situation is abusive and it probably is killing me. But I am sure, deep down, he or she really needs me and loves me. What would they do without me?" Then there is the victim, of the "I can't" dragon who whispers a spell—of two words only. "I can't, I can't, I can't." When I ask such patients if they can take responsibility for their health, I hear "I can't, I can't stop smoking, I can't make a difference, I can't lose weight, I can't eat healthy, I can't exercise, move, change my relationship, get another job, go back to school" etc., etc. This chant is usually intoned with a long-suffering whine and it's the echo of the twin dragons of hopelessness and despair. If you get sucked into their lair, it can be a long, hard climb back out. Taking a head count of the inhabitants of the shadow is rather like performing a role call of the deadly sins. No wonder it is a place we try to avoid. But we shun it at our own peril, for the road to healing runs straight through it. Besides, there is that treasure I spoke of earlier.

Deep in the shadow there is a prize. It is a prize so precious that it is defended by many fire-breathing monsters circling around it. Valued beyond all material wealth, the acquisition of this prize means the difference between inner life satisfaction and inner death. The treasure is nothing less than our connection with the life-force itself; it is our vitality, our wholeness and our love. I call this the "holy grail." To claim the prize, we must be prepared to penetrate the heart of darkness—the land of the shadow. This is not a journey for the faint-hearted. It takes courage, patience and perhaps many acts of heroism. Certainly, there will be dragons to be slain, tricked or lulled to sleep. It is the very hardest of work but it is definitely worth the effort.

How Do I Navigate in the Shadow?

How then do we wind our way in and out of the maze-like corridors deep in the shadow to arrive at our prize? This journey, certainly, was never taught to me in school or even in my postgraduate training. Although psychotherapy is one way to explore the shadow, for some of you this may not be the answer. For some of us, the dragon of negative bias towards therapy forces us to convince ourselves that this is not the way. For others, the investment of time and money is far too great a burden to take on. But there is one place we can all turn to. It is the wellspring of myths, legends and fairy tales.

Many of these stories are instructive. They may serve as symbolic or psychological road maps to the darkest side of the psyche. Fortunately, we live in a time that has witnessed a rich resurgence in story-telling and the reawakening of interest in its meaning. Joseph Campbell and Robert Bly are recent proponents. Other powerful clarifiers of myth and archetype are Marion Woodman, Marie Louise Von Franz and Carl Jung. They direct pathways through the shadow and the road to the treasure. They also help teach us how to get back out again, a very important element in any successful quest. The precise paths and exact nature of the treasure will be slightly different for each pilgrim. But the trip is always interesting and worthwhile. Let's examine just a few of the insights these old stories provide for us.

Of all the storytellers, I feel most connected to Robert Bly. I have been to many of Robert Bly's workshops and have particularly enjoyed his rituals for men. It is truly amazing how he commands an almost regimental-sized body of men, providing insight and strength—lifting many men to peak experiences. In his workshops he recites poetry and tells stories. He beats drums and spits out teachings with incredibly wise meanings in a squeaky voice, full of humor. I will never forget his discussion of how little boys learn to see men through the eyes of their mothers. When a boy learns about his father through the eyes of his mother, his impression obviously can be distorted. Let me tell you one of Bly's stories. This is the story of Iron John.

In this tale, a boy loses a golden ball that he has been playing with. It falls into a lake. Now, in stories such as these, a golden ball does not necessarily mean the boy's parents were financially well-off, although in this case they were. The golden ball symbolizes the integration of the personality, a wholeness which the boy has lost. He is unable to retrieve the ball himself. The only one who can help him is Iron John, a wild man imprisoned in a cage. In order to free Iron John so the ball can be retrieved, the boy has to steal the key to the cage from his mother's room. To make matters worse, the key is located under her pillow. But, good boys don't do such things. And, as long as our young hero remains bound to being a good boy, he can forget about forming an alliance with his wild man, integrating the paradoxical elements of his personality and attaining a state of wholeness. Fortunately, the boy's longing to retrieve what he has lost overpowers the need to be his mother's good boy. He steals the key, frees the wild man and forms a mutually beneficial relationship with him. He thus regains his golden ball (his true self) and goes off into the woods with Iron John in search of new experiences, presumably things his mother would not approve of.

The moral of this story is not that we should fail to honor our mothers and fathers. Certainly, I am not suggesting that. But, part of the growing-up process involves separating ourselves from parental expectations. It is, after all, our lives we are living, not theirs. Unhappily, many people fail to make this separation and stay bound to parental energies, plans and dreams, often in a state of seething, albeit unconscious resentment. The energy that should have gone into the development of the adult becomes locked into the shadow instead. And, energies trapped in the shadow never see the light or grow up. They stay childish, even infantile, as does that part of an individual's personality. Good boys do not grow up to be good men. They really don't grow up at all. The dragons have sucked their growth energy into the caverns below.

As a cardiologist, I see a lot of "good boys" with heart disease. In my workshops I have learned that they carry around a lot of denial about anger—especially toward the women in their lives—or the ones that hide the keys to the wild man's cage under their pillows. Let me tell you about the case of Tim.

Tim came in for therapy following an extensive cardiological evaluation for chest pain. Fortunately, all of his tests were normal. He had a history of resting and exertional chest pain and considerable fear about the possibility of heart disease. As a young boy, he had witnessed his father having a nonfatal heart attack at the age of 34. Although Tim was resistant in the first few sessions, he had considerable awareness that his chest pain had a lot to do with the feelings of heartbreak that he experienced as a young child. At the time of his therapy, his marriage was in trouble. He was experiencing little emotion and was suffering from a low-grade depression. He also lived in constant fear of dying. The initial period of his therapy focused on his hurt as a child. He was the youngest of four children. His childhood was full of criticism and lack of love and acceptance. He admitted to being very lonely. In order to get approval for love, Tim became a good boy, sacrificing anger and all his negative feelings. As a good boy, he did the chores and the yard work, folded his clothes, counseled and listened to his mother. He recalled that his mother had constantly corrected him in toilet training. He was always told that he was a very, very good boy.

In therapy, Tim had memories of being terrorized by his father and mother's behavior. His parents split up on numerous occasions and frequently argued in the presence of the children. Although Tim did see his father on occasion, he felt no real closeness to him. Tim's recollection of his mother was one of horror and disgust. He described her as having a "ghoulish quality." In therapy, he also sensed the strong possibility of an incestual relationship between them. Tim described his mother as sad, depressed and unavailable to him. Although he had felt sorrow for her, he felt that he had needed her and, as any little boy would, wanted to care for her and make her feel good. Since his mother had been beaten by his father, Tim could not really experience any negative feeling toward her. His mother also forbade him to express anger because this was "acting like your crazy father." The inability to express anger and rage as a child left him with considerable guilt, which was eventually reflected in his lack of sexual feeling.

At age four, he swallowed a bottle of aspirin as a suicidal gesture and made the false connection that "illness will buy me affection."

At around that time, this feeling was reinforced when his father was hospitalized with a heart attack. Throughout his childhood, Tim continued to avoid feeling. He did not cry and he held in his anger. If he experienced true feeling, he had the fear that his father would kill him. Thus, he ran the risk of full rejection by his mother and annihilation by his father. In therapy, however, he learned that he stored an enormous amount of rage in his body.

He related two stories of loss of control and rage. On one occasion, he flung a cat across the room in a fit of rage. Another time, during a karate class, he "almost killed someone" as a result of losing his composure. In therapy, he was able to admit to his rage and held-in anger. He did this by kicking on a mattress and using the words "why?" After experiencing this tremendous anger he admitted that some passion was reawakened in his marital relationship. Communication with his wife improved and he was able to experience more sexual feeling. The more anger Tim experienced, the better he felt. It gave him a true sense of strength and a feeling of being alive and free. By alienating his "unacceptable" energy and judging it negatively, Tim had believed that his anger was demonic, like a "monster" inside of him. By confronting his dragon, Tim regained his power and therefore was able to rechannel his energies into more positive directions.

Before body therapy, Tim's body was tight, coiled and rigid, reflecting his lack of feelings. His voice was constricted and at times high-pitched. The illusion of power and control was visible in his overinflated chest and his shallow mechanical way of breathing. His pectoral muscles were heavily armored to protect the heart. All were great cover-ups for the great sorrow and anguish that he experienced as a child. His waist was tight and contracted, and he admitted to little sexual feeling. His hostility towards women was locked in severe tensions of the upper back. His musculature was prominent, however, and his shoulders rounded as if he were burdened by women. The source of Tim's guilt was his inability to feel angry toward a helpless, pathetic mother. His underlying deep fear of women led to his fear of castration and, therefore, to the absence

of sexual feeling. Although he consciously admitted to having tremendously low self-esteem, feeling unlovable and mentally and
sexually inadequate, Tim's body had the stance, "I can take it."
Even though his father was the president of a large corporation,
Tim's Oedipal situation surfaced and he had the idea that he could
do better than his father. Fortunately for Tim, bioenergetic therapy
opened up feeling and awareness. With body work and bioenergetic
maneuvers to open his chest, he quickly broke into sobbing.

Crying released some of his tension. Although he always felt better after crying, he frequently had episodes of intense chest and
arm pain following his sessions. Tim also had difficulty in utilizing
his voice in therapy. Frequently I needed to extend his neck and
open up the throat. Soft pressure on the diaphragm enabled his
voice to break through and release feeling. At times, his soft cries
had an anguished quality.

The avoidance of the pain of reopening the hurt child's
heart to release feeling is perhaps the greatest resistance any
patient can offer a therapist. Tim did not really want to examine the pain. He did not want to get in touch with the feelings
of heartbreak he had experienced as a child. As a child he had
felt that he could die. In therapy, he was confronted with a
seemingly life-threatening dilemma by reexamining such feeling. By utilizing the voice, he was able to break through into
deep emotion. His hostility towards women was expressed by
hitting and striking a mattress with his fists. By using the
words "leave me alone," and by connecting the voice with
the hitting motions of his arms, Tim was able to get into true,
deep anger. At times, his anger assumed a theatrical quality.
As his therapist, I felt as if he were testing me with his anger
and rage. He feared that I would abandon or annihilate him.
This was the re-enactment of his childhood.

Tim's lack of sexual responsiveness to his wife seemed like
an expression of his hostility towards and fear of women.

Unable to get back at his mother, he retaliated by withholding sexual feeling from his wife. And his unconscious negative feeling towards women was expressed in an inability to give himself fully to sexual pleasure with her. His premature ejaculation was a manifestation of his deep pelvic tension. Tim was engaged in a power struggle with his wife on two levels—sex and business. Although he felt inferior to his wife on a sexual level, he felt even more castrated economically—since she was making more money than he was. As a boy, he felt powerless with his mother, and as a man he felt powerless with his wife. After having repressed his memory of those experiences with his mother, he reexperienced feeling powerless and sexually inadequate with his spouse. As Tim worked through his unconscious conflicts, he realized that his wife, like his mother, was cold and critical. When he realized that he had chosen a wife like his mother, he abruptly ended the marriage.

Thus, Tim's fear of love and his mistrust of women can be traced back to the experience of heartbreak that he suffered as a small child. In trying to find love, he set up a vicious cycle. Tim wanted women to love him; however, he could not reach out for love or experience it. He wanted his mother to love him. He wished his wife would love him. He spent his whole life trying to have people love him. Although he wanted to be in a relationship with a woman and wanted a woman to need him, when a woman found him attractive and had feeling for him, he then hated her for it. This powerful unconscious negative transference had a tremendous impact on both his psychological and physical life. The psychic pain of his heartache and heartbreak manifested itself in a frozen chest prone to chest pain.

For all practical purposes, Tim possessed a coronary-prone personality. On the surface, as an engineer, he was aggressive, ambitious and successful. But on a deeper level, his painful experience of rejection and subsequent fear of love placed undue stress upon his heart. Is Tim prone to cardiac illness?

Will Tim fulfill the family tradition and face the same demise as his father who recently died of congestive heart failure? The answer to these questions is probably not. Although Tim has the family history, personality, character type and drive associated with coronary heart disease, the fact that he is feeling the pain of heartbreak and experiencing his depression and despair probably protect him from the perils of this disease. The mobilization of his anger and the release of his deep sadness through crying and sobbing alleviated the tensions associated with heartbreak and freed him from the path to heart disease. In a therapeutic relationship, he is encouraged to express these profound shadow feelings and thus experience his true self.

The case of Tim illustrates the shadow emotions that reside in every one of us. That is, Tim represented the "good boy," the one with the smile which covered up his intense anger and rage. In my practice of cardiology, I have encountered many men who have come to see me with problems of impotence. In order for a man to really own his sexuality, he has to own his anger, particularly that connected with the women who are closest to him. For many men impotence is displaced anger toward women. Although many of my male patients have disagreed with me, some of them, in workshops as well as individual therapy, have grown to appreciate the grip that suppressed anger has on them and their sexuality. Through therapy, many of my patients have also gotten in touch with the many other shadow emotions that have a strange hold on our lives.

Another creature lurking in our shadow, which we often encounter in fairy tales and myths, is the big, bad, hungry wolf. The wolf is an archetype for an insatiable, psychoemotional vortex that nothing can ever fill. We find it most fully manifested in those who are "relentlessly" needy. In the words of Von Franz, "if one is kind to them, they demand more and more. Give such people an hour, a week and they will want two. If you give them two, they will want three. They want to see you in your spare time and if you give them that, they will want to marry you, and if you married them, they would want to eat you. They are completely driven." This creature of the shadow reflects that in every one of us there is something small and frightened yearning to be loved. These are hungry wolves that drain our energies, and seem to have a deep sense of alienation as the cornerstone of their foundation. They arise from a sense of neither belonging in the world or to it. It seems that they can never have or do or be enough in life to safeguard their own survival. Life in such a context is a ceaseless, exhausting struggle. Many will go to extremes to fulfill their incessant desire to be needed.

We now come to the "ring of power," one of the symbols of the shadow which is, in reality, the opposite of the wolf. The ring of power confers the ability to dominate. Whoever holds the ring has absolute power and control. It's a prize that's hotly pursued, not only in fairy tales, but in our professional and personal dramas. Power and control are deep shadow emotions that afflict every coronary-prone personality. The need to control crushes the life out of our soul. No one states this more clearly than Tolkein in his *Lord of the Rings* trilogy. Through these volumes, the author delineates how obsession, possession and the cold but passionate will to power spread darkness through the land. It is a good metaphor for the way in which such ugly psychological demons cast darkness across the unconscious. In the end, freedom from this evil is possible only through a sacrifice of great price. Balance is restored, but no one is left unscathed. Harmony, love and health cannot coexist beside the will to power, the need to control. They can only flourish when control is relinquished through an act of surrender. This act of surrender is often the final task required of us before we can bring our lives and our energies out of the captivity of the shadow. It is a frightening step, but a vital one. Not everyone will be able to do it, and those who cannot will remain, at least in part, forever captive and forever lost.

One way of surrendering is to become catastrophically ill, such as by having a heart attack. Catastrophic illness literally forces one to surrender. The heart is, indeed, the king of the body. The heart will not only tell you the truth, it will force you to see the truth. And if you don't listen to its message, you could die. The need to be in control can indeed be a deadly dragon. I have discussed some of the many demons and dragons lurking in our shadow: anger, rage, neediness, control and greed are all components of our personalities. But they don't have to be our fate. Our vast collection of fairy tales, stories, myths and legends can offer us tremendous insight and guide us through the metaphorical land of the shadow. There are also a variety of body-oriented techniques that can be used to mobilize the energies held within the shadow. If you can express some of these emotions, you can modify any of your emotional states.

Mobilizing the Energies in the Shadow

I consider anger the Achilles heel of heart disease. We must be in touch with this emotion if we are going to heal our hearts. But, for many of us, the pattern is to deny the anger, disown it and drive it underground where it gradually metamorphasizes into rage. Rage is the ugliest of all emotions because it is uncontrolled anger which can be dangerous to ourselves as well as to others. Most of us are reluctant to give in to our rage out of the fear that we may lose control and hurt ourselves or someone else. Let me tell you about Phil.

The case of Phil, a near-death resulting from aortic dissection, reveals the deadly impact of internal, unreleased rage. Phil was a World War II veteran who managed to donate approximately 18 gallons of blood to the Red Cross. His blood pressure was taken on all of these occasions and it had never been found to be high. He also had a respectable cholesterol level and was a nonsmoker. He had a low stress profile and a low-stress job managing a nursing home. But tragedy hit one day.

Since economic conditions were bad, the owner/supervisor of the nursing home summoned him into the office and asked him to fire his best nurse. A quarrel followed. He described his feelings of intense rage and said that he had "wanted to kill" his boss. Instead, Phil held in his rage. As things started to quiet down, the owner/supervisor then asked Phil to drive him to the airport. This was the last straw. He felt abused, helpless and controlled. Unable to express his rage, Phil turned it inward. He suddenly felt a pain in his left shoulder and became pale and diaphoretic. He collapsed. The nurse whom he was supposed to fire took his blood pressure and found it to be 70/0. She then frantically drove him to the emergency room. Fortunately, I was there seeing another patient when he arrived. Although he was barely alive, a quick diagnosis of dissection of the aorta was made and he was transferred to a tertiary hospital where he spent approximately 12 hours in surgery for repair of his torn aorta.

I eventually went to court for this man, representing him in a worker's compensation case to testify that his aortic dissection was the direct result of acute emotional stress related to his boss's behavior. I later reported his story in the medical literature, illustrating the powerful impact of unreleased rage and anger. Phil was not in touch with his tremendous anger; he was totally unaware; and he amost died from this denial of what was really happening to his body.

Internalized anger which leads to rage can culminate in disaster. Therefore, it is necessary to release bits and pieces of anger before it evolves into to uncontrolled rage. But anger does not have to be an ugly emotion. There is an energy in anger that, when channeled correctly, can be utilized as a powerful healing force. Some of my patients who have been through painful and frightening experiences get angry, sometimes even taking it out on me because I at times cannot just "fix them." When I see their strong, angry feelings coming through, however, I support these feelings, saying to them "now you are getting better and fighting back." People with cancer, heart disease or any life-threatening illness need to channel their emotions in a way that gives them strength, clarity and purpose.

When you are in touch with and release the feelings of anger, you will be able to feel the emotion and, most importantly, you will be able to identify what it is doing to your body. Do you have "looks that could kill?" Do you strike out verbally or physically? Do you flare your nostrils in a fit of anger? Do you become impatient to the point of interrupting others? Or do you turn your anger against yourself and become depressed? It is helpful to track the pattern of this emotion in your body language.

Some of my patients need to express their anger in a physical way and have asked me for guidance in how to do this. In our Healing the Heart workshops, we perform many expressive exercises with anger.

Learning to say "no," setting a boundary with real feeling is a crucial step in the right direction. The ability to say "no" and stand by it is one of the hallmarks of a secure and grounded person. Other exercises may include using the voice to verbally express negativity, jutting out the jaw, making a fist and using arm motions such as striking out or hitting. Even letting yourself go into a temper tantrum can release withheld feeling, resulting in a general relaxation of the body. Exercises such as these loosen up spasticity and chronic tension, especially in the upper back and neck. Kicking and hitting can be used as a form of protest to mobilize underlying fears of hurt and anger. Frequently, in workshop situations, I will ask a patient to lie down on the mattress and kick, perhaps 100 to 200 times.

Repeating the words "why" or "no" often adds vocal feelings of protest which heighten the experience. The triad of expression, breathing and feeling allows the patient to make more contact with himself during these maneuvers. Another exercise that I frequently do in group situations is to ask a participant to stand in front of a mattress with various pillows on it. He or she is asked to breathe deeply and strike the pillows with their fists after raising their hands high over their head with back arched. Such maneuvers release energy from both the upper body, pelvis and upper thighs. This, in essence, is bringing your whole body into the anger exercise. By using the voice, striking with the fists and arching the back, the participant can enter "wholeheartedly" into the exercise. Such exercises energetically bring emotions to the surface, the principle underlying bioenergetic analysis. I will be talking more about the principles of bioenergetic therapy in a subsequent chapter on healing the heart. Although doing one or two exercises is not going to release you completely, performing these maneuvers over time will assist the body in discharging chronic tension. These exercises can also be adapted to access rage, sadness, lust and any other emotional state you have been keeping under wraps. Once an emotion has been accessed and expressed, this energy becomes more available for healthy understanding and reintegration.

When dealing with the contents of the shadow, you simply need to come to terms with the fact that if you are human, you have a shadow and it is filled with things of which you are not proud. But once you are in touch with your feelings, impulses and desires, you own them. You spend less time and energy pretending they are not there. You live less in denial and spend more time grounded in the truth of the body. You learn to honor your energies instead of repressing them. When you own your anger, you become less defensive. When you own your fear, you become less anxious. When you learn to understand the source of your hatreds, you become less prejudiced. Remember, the taller a tree grows, the more deeply it must plunge its roots into the earth. The more fully an individual grows or expands, the more completely he must examine his own depths. Otherwise, we will wind up like a forest of top-heavy hemlocks. These lovely trees send their roots out broadly but not deeply. Any strong wind can blow them over. It is not a way of life I would choose for myself or recommend to my patients. Be aware that when repressed negative feelings implode, or explode, the results can raise havoc with your heart, your health, your relationships and even your life. But, it doesn't have to come to that. By owning your shadow and learning your interior landscape, you will learn to accept those things in yourself that, at first, may have seemed unacceptable.

Remember, the shadow will still be there whether you own it or not. A heart attack or a serious illness will bring you face to face with it. The question you must consider is whether you will take this message as an opportunity for exploration, adventure or quest. If you wait, you may be dragged along the road in a forced march. In my own life I have tried both approaches. The quest is a far better choice. The final gift of such an experience is that it teaches us to embrace our own humanity, with all our limitations, flaws and physical mortality. When we can embrace these qualities in ourselves, we are able to embrace the humanity of others and become, in the process, more embraceable as well.

The path through the shadow inevitably leads us back into the light and leads us into greater life and deeper joy than we were capable of knowing before the journey. Unleashing the power trapped within the emotional negativity of our "shadow" creates a space within the heart conducive for loving. After this journey through the shadow, we are now able to investigate some of the ways to heal the heart.

CHAPTER 7

———— ✦ ————

Healing the Heart

My traditional training in cardiology enabled me to feel highly competent in what I was doing, but on a deeper level, I knew that I was not completely fulfilled in my work. Something was missing in my role as a physician and healer. As the continual battle against illness began to take its toll, I searched for the missing links in the quest for healing. But, it was not until I began my training as a psychotherapist that I began to appreciate the deeper process in which health is maintained, lost, regained—and often lost again.

Previously I mentioned that pathology is really a form of "dis-ease" that emerges from a chaotic imbalance between the energies of mind, body and spirit. To embrace this trinity is to embrace the heart as the ultimate organ of pulsating muscle, engaging the energies and interactions of mind, body and spirit. After all, whatever one thinks affects what one feels. And whatever one feels affects the heart rate: how fast the heart beats and how well the heart pumps. As we have noted, fear, the most visceral of all emotions, causes the heart to beat rapidly and forcefully. Fear may cause palpitations, pounding or irregularity of the heartbeat, which is sensed as considerable distress by the person. Anyone who has experienced a panic reaction will tell you that their greatest fears originate from the rapid and overwhelming sensations in the heart. Sometimes the heart may beat in such an erratic fashion that it causes great worry and stress for the individual. When this happens, vigilant "conversations" develop between the heart and the mind.

Love may also cause an increase in heart rate and pumping action, but the effects of love are experienced as nurturing forces. Ask anyone who has ever been in love and he or she will tell you that the heart beats faster when seeing, embracing or even thinking about the beloved. Correlated with such positive emotion, the awareness of the heartbeat is overshadowed by the pleasurable anticipation of excitement and passion. Remember that the heart is under the control of both the brain and the autonomic nervous system. To review, the autonomic system is divided into two complementary but opposite branches, the sympathetic and parasympathetic arms.

Sympathetic and Parasympathetic Nervous Systems

The sympathetic nervous system (SNS) responds acutely and chronically to external stressors, resulting in ways to "protect" the organism. The release of inhibited power and the mobilization of energy may be expressed as aggression, negativity, struggle or a fight/flight response. When the SNS is suddenly activated, aggressive energy is mobilized and discharged, allowing an individual to quickly return to a state of balance. But when the SNS activation becomes chronic, the contained energy is not fully discharged. This often happens in our modern day tug-of-war between personal life demands and social constraints, causing the body to become trapped in a continual state of "sympathetic overdrive." The price the body pays for holding this state includes increased muscle tension and contraction as well as energetic blocks leading to disease in the forms of high blood pressure and heart disease.

As discussed earlier, parasympathetic activation, on the other hand, allows for softening, expanding and letting down, components of Wilhelm Reich's model of expansion and contraction. According to Reich, the parasympathetic nervous system (PNS) operates in the direction of expansion, "out of self toward the world," including pleasure and joy. Reich views the sympathetic nervous system as operating in the direction of contraction "away from the world into the self," often leading to contraction and displeasure. We live in a continuous alteration between expansion and contraction. This is the paradoxical nature of the sympathetic nervous system. In an emergency, the SNS can mobilize our energies; it can save our lives. At the same time, chronic activation of the SNS from daily stressors has the potential to harm us. It is the imbalance in polarities between expansion and contraction or energy-saving processes versus energy-spending processes that affect the very essence of energy flow and pulsation. This can be a chronic source of *"dis-ease."*

What factors impede cellular pulsation and block energy flow within the human body? In heart disease, there appear to be several culprits leading to the imbalanced oxygenation of the cells lining the coronary arteries. Oxidative changes may occur through harmful breathing patterns, inadequate or self-destructive eating habits and stress. Beliefs and attitudes often underlie the physiological changes and body armoring associated with chronically withheld emotions. The health of the body begins to deteriorate when its physical, emotional and mental processes become dis-integrated and fail to work in harmony.

To establish health and balance, the fragmented parts of the self must be reintegrated by including proper nutrition and exercise as well as psychotherapeutic and spiritual components. Psychotherapeutic techniques are directed toward the release of painful emotion and past trauma. Encouraging play and laughter can enhance energy. Both dynamic and bioenergetic releasing exercises are physical and energetic components essential in healing the heart. The ultimate goal of reintegration of body, mind and spirit is the reopening of the heart to love and the development of a spiritual connection. Now let's analyze all these channels, beginning with physical exercise.

Exercise

Regular exercise has been consistently demonstrated to strengthen the heart and circulatory system as well as build stamina and improve state of mind. Exercise can increase levels of endorphins in the body, leading to a feeling of well-being. This is frequently referred to as the "runner's high," a fact documented by scientific evidence.

However, there are many myths about exercise. The first myth is the "no pain, no gain" theory. You don't really need to break a sweat, jog, run or pump iron. Often my patients ask me what is the best form of exercise. I always give them the same answer. The best form of exercise is one that you will do with satisfaction and enjoyment. In my opinion, the two best forms of exercise are simple, pleasant and fun. I recommend walking and dancing.

Most of us don't think of walking and dancing as exercise, so think of these actions as "movement." Fifteen minutes of movement, at least two times a day, gives your heart and circulatory system the nurturing it needs.

If you can walk a mile or more once or twice a day, your heart will receive an adequate cardiovascular workout. I don't recommend jogging or running. These activities have many potential side effects such as ankle injuries, shin splints, hip problems and even rare incidences of sudden death. Though the American Heart Association recommends that you "run for your life," I have long disagreed with this statement. Although exercise has many established benefits, too much of the wrong kind of exercise can be harmful to your health. There are many cases on record, for example, of fatal heart attacks precipitated from some form of exercise. This has even occurred in marathon runners. From what we hear about the value of exercise, one would expect regular intensive running to have tremendous benefits for the heart. In certain ways it does, but we have to ask this question; "Why do some long-distance runners and athletes develop severe coronary heart disease?"

This fact had long been my concern until I reviewed the cardiological literature which focuses on this mystery. In an article published in *The American Journal of Cardiology* several years ago, the authors analyzed several runners who died while participating in races. Autopsy results of this study revealed that runners who had experienced sudden death had severe coronary heart disease similar to the hearts of people who have symptoms and suffer fatal heart attacks due to severe arteriosclerotic heart disease. The question we need to ask is whether or not these runners had been truly asymptomatic. Could they have had symptoms but denied them? I believe this type of scenario is typical of individuals such as Jim Fixx who died while running. The problem for contemporary cardiologists, like myself, is that although many exercising people have severe arteriosclerotic heart disease, they are not at all aware of it. They are not "in touch" either because they deny symptoms they do feel or really don't *feel* the symptoms. It is a fact that 90 percent of severe coronary heart disease is asymptomatic. That is why it is so crucial not to think of exercise as magical risk-free protection or as a cure for your heart.

Instead, I want you to view exercise as you would a drug. It has great potential benefits when it is used properly and in the right dosages. But exercise can be hazardous if overdone or abused.

Here are a few cautions about strenuous exertion. If you are a sedentary type of individual with little or no regular exercise program and you suddenly engage in some intensive

exertion such as changing a flat tire, picking up a TV or pushing a car, you may be especially vulnerable to a heart attack.
We have all known someone who has suffered a heart attack
during or after strenuous activity such as jogging, shoveling
snow, lifting something heavy or even after sexual activity.

The known correlation between heavy exertion and heart
attacks has been clarified by two recent studies in *The New
England Journal of Medicine.* These studies indicated that, although heavy physical exertion can trigger a heart attack, people who exercise regularly do have a reduced long-term risk
of coronary events after heavy exertion. However, these studies found that although heavy physical exertion was strongly
associated with an increased risk of heart attack, people who
did no regular exercise had a much higher relative risk of a
heart attack after unexpected bouts of heavy exertion. The
patients who exercised five times or more per week over a
long period of time had substantially lower relative rates of
heart attack triggered by strenuous exertion.

As a cardiologist, I feel it is important that you consider
regular exercise in your daily routine to strengthen and protect your heart. However, if you are a sedentary "couch po-
tato" and you are suddenly required to engage in vigorous
exertion, your risk of heart attack is much higher than the risk
of someone who exercises daily. For this reason I recommend
walking and dancing as enjoyable forms of rhythmic daily
exercises. With these activities, you can safely provide considerable protection for your heart, especially if you are required
to perform unexpected bouts of physical activities.

It is important to walk and dance regularly but not inten-
sively. Remember, when you walk and dance, you are expressing movement with your body. Remind yourself to breathe
during these activities. By breathing deeply, your movement
will become easier as well as more pleasant. It is also important to pay attention to how your body feels. Many of my
patients report to me that they feel better and stronger after

they have walked or danced. Many patients report that walking is not only beneficial for their physical health, but their psychological well-being as well. Research has also demonstrated that individuals who report feeling better physically feel better emotionally as well. There are many ways you can incorporate walking into your life.

First, look around to see where you can add extra walking to your daily activities. For example, I incorporate walking into my life by avoiding elevators. I walk up and down the stairs. When I park my car at the hospital, I park it in the most distant corner of the parking lot. In this way, I walk further and enjoy it. I also recommend that you walk your dog. It is important not only for your physical well-being, but for your dog's as well. Making a connection with an animal is truly conducive to healing. And always consider walking instead of driving short distances for errands or visits. When you walk, remember to take in the scenery, breathe deeply, smell the air, look at the clouds, the sun, the moon and the stars. Take it all in.

I remember several years ago, I was walking with Dr. Alexander Lowen at an International Conference on Bioenergetic Analysis. As we were walking, he asked me if I were paying attention to my body. He encouraged me to notice if I was feeling my hips and legs as well as my chest. He reminded me how important it is to make walking an enjoyable activity. You, too, should pay particular attention to your hip movement. Try to loosen your hips. You'll feel yourself move more smoothly. From this point you may get in touch with the ebb and flow of motion in the rest of the body. Walking can be so magical! One of the things I like to do when I walk is just daydream, letting my imagination run freely.

Walking is also a great way to relieve stress, think about new ideas and review what is going on in your life. I like to use walking not only as a form of exercise, but also as a way to escape. As automatic as brushing your teeth, I suggest you incorporate at least a mile or two a day of walking into your daily schedule. If you are unable to do it regularly every day, then try every other day. If it is raining, snowing, too hot or too cold, try walking in a large indoor mall. Or if you prefer to walk in your home, try using a treadmill. And remember, walking can be done at any age.

Recently, I was in New Brunswick, Canada on a fishing trip with a few of my friends. My guide was 75 years old. Not only did he have abundant knowledge of the salmon habitat in the river, but he was also in great physical and emotional shape. He walked with me up and down the river, around rocks, up and down boulders. We also walked in fast-moving water. I was absolutely impressed with this man's physical and emotional well-being. Like Zorba the Greek, he put his "whole heart" into guiding me. Although I was 26 years younger than my comrade, I sensed that he was in as good, if not better, physical condition than I. For him, walking is a major component of his life. He told me that he was also an avid dancer.

Many of my patients think I am joking when I first tell them that they should dance for exercise. I am still not sure why. Maybe it is because most people think of dancing as something reserved only for special occasions like weddings, parties or nights out. Most of us hear music every day and we probably should instinctively and unconsciously respond to it. You see, I believe that music affects us on a deep, sometimes unconscious level. Oftentimes we can't explain why we respond to certain music or even describe what it is about. For example, some of us have pleasant memories when we listen to waltzes or concertos. For many of us, music in ranges of 60 to 80 beats per minute reminds us of a previous pleasant experience. That experience may be from our origins in the womb.

It is an established fact that unconsciously many of us prefer music in these ranges. A growing baby is accustomed to her mother's heartbeat. If the experience in utero was a good one, the baby remembers the beating of the mother's heart, which is usually between 60 to 80 beats per minute. Later on in life this tempo can create feelings of joy and euphoria when listening to music that reminds us of this previous experience. This is why some people love to dance to soft music.

Think back to the last time you danced. I hope it wasn't too long ago. Think about how you felt on both physical and emotional levels. Remember, when you put a lot of energy into dancing, moving around and using your arms and legs at the same time, you are giving your body a physical workout. Dancing is aerobic because it increases the oxygenation of your body. The exercise of dancing is also coupled with an emotional benefit. Many feelings and emotions may come up when you dance, especially with ballroom dancing. Dancing can also be a great tension release. Some dances, like the tango, are full of feeling. As a young boy, I used to love to watch my father and mother dance. Dancing can have a tremendous graceful quality to it. And when you put your heart into it and close your eyes your negative feelings slowly diminish. Think about it, how can you fully put your heart into dancing and feel negative at the same time? It is just not possible.

Another great benefit of dancing as an exercise is that it also gives you permission to express your sexuality in a socially acceptable way. For example, in many types of dancing your hips are involved. I love to dance with the Brazilians because they dance with such feeling and intensity. We all hold a lot of tension in our hips, pelvis, lower back and the long muscles of our legs. I know that when I let myself completely go while dancing, my chronic lower back pain oftentimes just disappears. And remember, there is also another tremendous benefit of dancing. It allows you to make contact with others. When you dance, you make intimate contact with your spouse or your friend. It is that kind of contact and closeness that helps heal your heart.

Dancing and walking are truly the most important exercises to consider. However, in the overall framework of healing your heart, there are other nontraditional types of exercises, the so-called bioenergetic exercises that can literally "open the chest." These exercises facilitate the flow of energy out of the thoracic cage as well as release energy in many of the segments of the body that are blocked or stagnant. Before beginning bioenergetic exercises, let me review bioenergetic analysis.

Bioenergetics

Bioenergetics is a body-oriented analytic therapy that focuses upon muscular tension in the body and the physical expression of emotional conflict in the personality. The practice of bioenergetic analysis includes improving the flow of energy in the body, including the energy of the heart. This is achieved by increasing the individual's capacity to feel by resolving early character patterns and attitudes that have become structured in the body and interfere with its rhythmic and pulsatory movements. Through special movements, exercises and body positions, the patient in bioenergetic analysis gains deeper contact with his body. From awareness, insight, and contact, the patient in therapy begins to learn the relationship between his or her present physical state and the earlier experiences of infancy and childhood which contribute to it.

One goal of bioenergetic analysis is learning to breathe fully. Through the process of breathing, one can get more in touch with feeling. The expression of feeling allows the body to become more alive, thus, increasing its life force. When one realizes such natural pulsatory movements of the total body, the health of the heart also increases.

According to Alexander Lowen, when working with the body, a bioenergetic therapist needs to be aware of two principles:

1. Any limitation of motility and pulsation is both the result and cause of emotional difficulties arising from unresolved infantile conflict. It is the *persistence* of such tension that creates emotional difficulties that place stress in our adult lives.

2. Any restriction of natural respiration is both the result and cause of early emotional conflict. Such anxiety in childhood situations disturbs natural respiration. If the anxiety-producing situation persists and is prolonged, the disturbance of respiration becomes structured in thoracic and abdominal tension. The inability to breathe freely under emotional stress is a frequent experience of the tension and anxiety of everyday life situations. Often the bioenergetic therapist will use breathing exercises during the course of a session. The way a client breathes may begin to tell a story about him or her.

Every physical expression of the body has a meaning. The quality of one's handshake, the posture, the look in the eyes, the tone of the voice, the movement of expression and the overall energy all convey important information. When these expressions become fixed and habitual, they tell a story of earlier experiences. The interpretation of this "past experience" adds a new dimension to the therapeutic experience of both client and therapist.

For example, patients in bioenergetic analysis can discover that their rigidities may be a defense against an overwhelming rage. As we know, such rage occurs from rejection. Given the opportunity to express rage by pounding, kicking and voicing negativity, the patient discovers that he or she will not be abandoned, annihilated or humiliated for expressing feelings. Through the acceptance of real feeling, the individual comes in contact with his body and other aspects of his reality.

Kicking and hitting can be used as a form of protest to mobilize underlying feelings of hurt and anger. By encouraging the

triad of breathing, feeling and expression, the bioenergetic therapist assists the client to "let it happen." By observing the natural
pulsatory movements of the body without interference, the bioenergetic therapist facilitates increased contact for the client
with himself as well as his feelings.

It is important to think energetically; energy flow is the
functional principle underlying bioenergetic analysis. The
most important factors determining health and illness, in reality, are the energy level an individual has and how available
that energy is to be utilized by the body. Many illnesses, in
bioenergetic terms, are the result of blocked energy. For example, in heart disease, we know that the energy block is in
the chest, diaphragm and the throat. One could say that in
colon cancer, energy is blocked in the gut. Stagnation of energy in the prostate may render one susceptible to prostate
cancer.

Muscular tensions and rigidities must also be viewed energetically. Muscular tension is a dynamic force. Since tensions
do not develop overnight, they cannot be released by a single
experience. Often a single tension pattern will require consistent work over a long period of time before it changes.

Bioenergetics frequently involves "hands-on work" between the therapist and the patient. It is the role of the therapist to assist the client to free up his or her stagnant energy.
Just as stagnant water becomes poisonous, stagnant energy in
the body can also become toxic. It is the goal of the patient
and the role of the therapist to help release these blocks. Frequently, the work creates exchanges of emotion known as
transference and countertransference. In bioenergetics they
occur as with any other form of psychotherapy. Transference
is defined as feelings that the client has towards the therapist.
Usually, the therapist represents the ideal mother or father.
Sometimes intense feelings are generated in the client. For
example, if the therapist "disappoints" the client in the therapy process, this may generate a charge of feeling or emotion

in the client. In transference, the emotional reaction to the therapist is often a reenactment of the client's childhood interaction with his or her parents.

Countertransference is defined as emotions provoked in the therapist by the client while encouraging him or her to focus on significant issues. At times the therapist needs to explore with the patient an issue that he or she has worked through in the past. This may create feelings in the therapist. Frequently, a good therapist will tell the patient what he is experiencing in his body as a way to explore his countertransference with the patient. Countertransference may also arise from bioenergetic exercises utilized to ease energetic blocks, enhance breathing and also bring out emotion. Such exercises are absolutely critical in releasing energy from chronic contraction, especially in the chest wall and even the heart.

BIOENERGETIC EXERCISES

The basic function of bioenergetic exercise is to free up the armoring process localized in various parts of the body. When energy is contracted, energetic pulsation is inhibited and a considerable amount of energy is consumed in the holding attitude. Armoring in the child is defensive and protective. In the adult this armoring can be destructive, as the rigidification of the chest wall creates a chronic ineffective utilization of energy. The holding is not necessarily limited to external muscles such as the visible muscles of the chest wall and body. Holding also creates ineffective utilization of energy occurring internally, such as in the deep pelvic muscles, diaphragm, lungs and even the heart itself. It is the release of both external and internal contracted energies that is so pivotal in healing the heart. The exercises must be organized in a way that can successfully interrupt the frozen energy or the armoring process in the body to enhance core pulsation and reestablish homeostasis. These are the key components of bioenergetic work.

The bioenergetic therapist uses several techniques to mobilize energy and breath. For example, the bioenergetic stool *(Figure 1)* devised by Alexander Lowen in the 1950's is a psychotherapeutic tool used by therapists to mobilize breathing. It is approximately 24 inches high. Usually a rolled up blanket is strapped to the top. The patient lies back on the stool with his arms stretched above his head. This is designed to open the chest, expand the diaphragm, and bring the breath into the belly. The client often feels a stretch from the pelvis to the neck.

Since most people have considerable tension in the muscles of the back, neck and diaphragm, this position may be quite uncomfortable. It should be used only under medical supervision, preferably with an experienced bioenergetic psychotherapist.

The primary function of the bioenergetic stool is to open up the breathing capacity of the chest. If the patient "holds" or blocks against opening up, he or she may begin to experience discomfort. The patient is encouraged to surrender, open the voice and focus on the breathing. As he or she does so, the pain usually disappears and feelings arise. The increase in breathing brings about an increase in feeling. Heavily armored, defensive people may have tremendous resistance to these feelings. The more a person is in touch with his or her own body, the stronger she identifies with her feelings. However, it is very difficult to hold one's breath while laying over the stool. Sometimes, one will cough or choke as a result of bronchial tension or the blocking of sadness in the throat. Frequently I will ask a patient to make a sustained sound to stimulate deeper breathing. The inability to use the voice in this capacity usually suggests considerable tension and rigidity in the chest wall and lungs.

It is not always necessary to use a bioenergetic stool as the major intervention. Many times, such a stool is not available or we are unable to work with a therapist. Lying on the floor using a rolled-up blanket may create a similar situation of

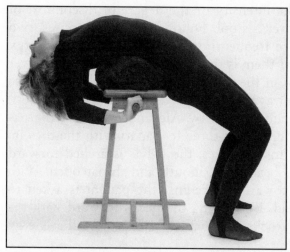

Figure 1.
Bioenergetic Stool

PHOTOGRAPHS BY
CARL McALLISTER

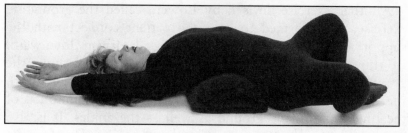

Figure 2. Cat Stretch

projecting the energy outward. For example, if you lay on the floor and stretch your body like a cat, the stretching of the arms and legs will bring out the energy of the chest and diaphragm, especially if you are breathing deeply. This will be further accentuated with a rolled-up blanket placed at the base of your spine. By pressing your buttocks into the floor and stretching the arms outward, the belly will lift. Not only will a maneuver like this create a tension-relieving stretch in the lower back and diaphragm, but it will also stimulate the movement of breathing *(Figure 2).*

Although the stretching and breathing process on the blanket roll is similar in technique to using a bioenergetic stool, it does not have the intensity or the degree of discomfort of working directly over a stool. Following these exercises, two other maneuvers are frequently used in balancing the energy of the body. One of them is the arch and bow. This maneuver relieves the tension in the lower back while at the same time displacing energy away from the pelvis, diaphragm and chest. In this exercise, again devised by Alexander Lowen, the patient stretches his feet about three feet apart with the toes in. With a little bend to the knees, the pelvis is arched forward with the belly out, head back, mouth and throat open. With the eyes pointing toward the ceiling, the patient is asked to sustain a long sound. By moving the pelvis forward with the hands on their buttocks, the patient can project the energy outward (Figure 3).

Another exercise devised by Lowen, called the grounding exercise, is performed to help the patient connect with the support of the ground. Here the energy is driven downward. In this exercise, the patient bends forward, touching the ground with his fingertips with the knees slightly bent. With the head bent down, the eyes should scan the soft touch of the fingertips on the ground as well as the ankles. It is also permissible to close the eyes in this exercise. The feet are about 12 to 18 inches apart and turned slightly inward. It is very important to have the patient drop his head loosely and to avoid cocking the head upward and outward.

In such a position, the patient assumes control. Actually when the head comes up spontaneously, it is a sure sign that a "will-to-power dragon" is lurking in the background. The purpose of the grounding exercise is to soften and let down. In this exercise, control is not the issue. This exercise is solely for making contact with the ground and feeling the support of your feet. As one holds the position for several minutes, the legs may begin to vibrate. It is the vibrations in the back of the legs that help relieve stress and tension in the pelvis and the extensor and flexor muscles of the upper and lower legs (Figure 4).

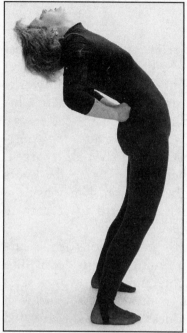

Figure 3. Arch and Bow

Figure 4. Grounding Exercise

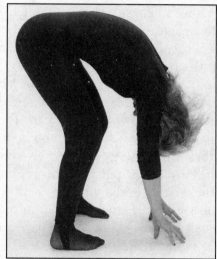

PHOTOGRAPHS BY
CARL McALLISTER

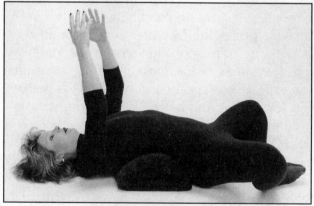

Figure 5.
Reaching with
Soft Arms

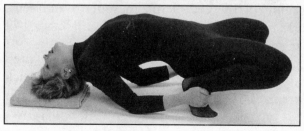
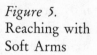

Figure 6.
Energizing
the Resistance

Another important technique to release feelings in the chest and to connect with the energy of the heart is simple reaching exercises. These are exercises I frequently use in group workshops, although they can also be used one-to-one. After bioenergetic exercises are used to facilitate and charge the energy of the body, I ask the patient to assume the reverse frog position. In this exercise, the lower back and pelvis are charged. The client presses both feet together and opens up the knees and pelvis as wide as she can. In this position, I may ask the client to move the legs slowly back and forth to accentuate vibrational energy in the pelvis and legs.

Many times, patients will report these sensations as pleasurable as the body vibrates with streaming energy down into the legs. This position is comfortable and often evokes softness. At times, I will ask patients to make soft sounds with their lips. Asking them to recall sadness or the loss of a loved one is frequently accompanied by crying and sadness. Having the patient reach with soft arms and adding a Gestalt maneuver where the patient places the face of a loved one in their hands may also evoke responses of sadness (Figure 5).

The expression of sadness is the most cleansing emotional expression we can experience. Crying uncontrollably is perhaps the best medicine for healing the heart. When crying emerges with deep sobs coming from the pelvis and belly, there is a tremendous release of energy in the diaphragm and heart. Almost any exercise using the arms is a way to indirectly connect with the heart. Remember my discussion of David Boadella's work in embryology in a previous analysis. Since the arms arise from the same region of the endoderm, mesoderm and ectoderm as the heart, simple arm motions are a subtle way of getting to the energy of the chest and heart.

Another more advanced exercise I use in "heavily armored" people is the bridge. The ability to say "no" is the hallmark of a grounded person. In bioenergetics, there is an old saying that you "can't say yes until you can say no." Ben Shapiro's exercise of "energizing the resistance" uses bridging as another way to take further risk and therefore create deeper surrender and opening. Many patients, for example, are totally resistant to any form of bioenergetic maneuvers. Sometimes their resistance is so strong that they cannot get anything from an exercise. When this happens, it is useful to energize that resistance by getting the patient to say "no" on both verbal and body levels. In the bridging exercise, the body is supported by the feet and the top of the head *(Figure 6)*.

The energy is projected upward and outward. Bridging opens the tops of the thighs, thus charging the feet, legs, chest, arms and eyes. Utilizing the voice with aggression and stretching the front of the body opens the throat. The aggressive nature of this exercise not only elicits feelings, but also stimulates breathing at the same time. Like work with the bioenergetic stool, however, this exercise should only be done with an experienced bioenergetic therapist.

There are other softening exercises that can be used to open the energy of the chest. Two exercises which I use frequently include lying down on the floor with the eyes open and directed toward the ceiling. One can use effortless arm and leg swings together in harmony to the right and left as a way to release the energy bound in the chest and pelvis. This exercise can be done alone or with a therapist. Another powerful exercise I have used often in group situations or in dyads, is having a "therapist" and "client" touch each other's breast plate or the center of the chest. In such a dyad, with one person facing the other, one can pull the left arm of the other, while placing the opposite hand in the center of the chest. The rhythmic flow between client and therapist together with the massaging motion of bone to bone contact of hand over chest is a useful maneuver for releasing energy from the chest. Frequently, just the touch of one's hand over the other's heart results in feelings of sadness. Such simple maneuvers allows one to "see" another. When you literally "touch another's heart" and make tender eye contact at the same time, you can see how vulnerable we all really are.

There are two other expressive exercises which are extremely helpful in mobilizing the energy of anger. In one exercise the patient brings the arms over the head with a slight arch to the back, propelling forward with a hitting motion. This can be done with one's fists or a tennis racket. The patient is also encouraged to let out sounds while hitting. This type of exercise is extremely useful in freeing up the tension in the upper back, neck and shoulders (Figure 7).

Another exercise which expresses the feeling of protest is the kicking exercise. In this exercise, the patient is asked to lay on a bed and do a scissor kick for approximately 100 to 200 times (Figure 8). The patient can do this on a mattress holding the sides of the mattress with his or her hands. During the kicking motion, the patient is frequently asked to loosen the head and shake it back and forth, thus giving up control. In addition, the words "no" or "why" can be shouted to elicit further emotion. My former mentor and teacher, Dr. Alexander Lowen, tells me that he kicks at least 200 times a day. After completing these expressive exercises, various other bioenergetic positions, including grounding and reaching, are frequently used as a way of "softening" the patient. Often during these maneuvers, patients may express feelings of sadness and vulnerability as they get more in touch with their breathing and feelings.

Although there are many more exercises we can use in bioenergetic analysis, these few maneuvers are essential in supporting the patient to open up the energy in various segments of the body with particular emphasis on the chest.

Breathing and Meditation

Breathing and mediation are two tools that will help bring about emotional healing as well as aid in reducing the stress and tension in our lives. For centuries, the bridge connecting

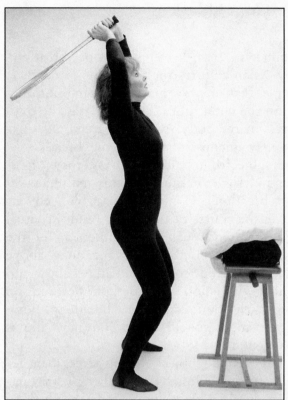

Figure 7.
The Hitting
Exercise

PHOTOGRAPHS BY
CARL McALLISTER

Figure 8.
The Kicking
Exercise

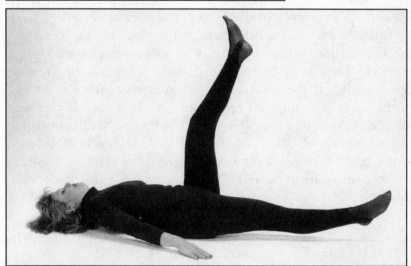

the body and the mind has been breathing. Proper breathing has been utilized by Asian cultures for thousands of years. It is known, for example, that diaphragmatic breathing not only reduces the tension in the chest, but it also increases the oxygen supply to the rest of the body. When we are afraid, anxious or nervous we may unconsciously hold our breath.

When people are subjected to chronic stress, they oftentimes become tense and rigid. Frequently, this tension takes the form of shallow breathing. Continued or prolonged improper breathing, over the course of time, may result in actual physical changes in the body such as rigidification of the upper body, chest and shoulders. High chest breathing, above the level of the diaphragm, tends to be rapid and shallow and is frequently associated with emotional upset, physical tension or mental stress. Slow, rhythmic abdominal breathing, however, is physiologically more suited to the body and allows greater intake of oxygen.

Proper breathing has been the subject of many stress management programs. In the fields of Gestalt psychotherapy, particularly bioenergetic therapy, deep breathing is used as a vehicle to loosen up the energy of the chest and to free emotions.

When we focus on breathing, we get out of the mind and back into the body. The best way to become aware of our need to breathe is to watch for signs of panic or anxiety. Frequently, in these situations we may want to eat, have a drink or even reach for a cigarette. Deep breathing is one way to get us through a crucial point when we might do something maladaptive and often self-destructive. Making contact with your body through your breath is an important way of reconnecting with yourself. Try this exercise of abdominal breathing.

Simple Abdominal Breathing

1. Lie on the floor and bend your knees.
2. Close your eyes.

3. Place your hands over your naval.
4. Breathe in through your nose.
5. Breathe out naturally and feel your abdomen fall beneath your hands.
6. Inhale a full deep breath and then exhale it completely.

Deep breathing can be practiced sitting or lying down. This type of deep breathing can be used to relieve emotional stress or, preventively, on a daily basis.

When you become comfortable with this exercise, try the "four breath" exercise which is a breathing exercise that I modified from Jean Achterberg and colleagues.

Sit comfortably with your back straight but relaxed.... focus on your breath and exhale and inhale three times.... then.... slowly.... begin to inhale ... As you feel the air moving in through your nose and down the back of your throat into your lungs, hear yourself saying deep inside yourself ... ONE.... feel the air moving back out.... as the next breath begins to fill your lungs, hear yourself saying.... TWO.... feel the air moving back out.... with the next breath in, hear yourself saying ... THREE.... feel the air moving back out.... with the breath, hear yourself saying.... FOUR.... feel the air moving back out.... repeat this cycle three times.... counting one to four with your breaths....

With each breath in.... feel your diaphragm moving down toward your feet.... and your lower abdomen beginning to expand.... with each breath out.... as your abdomen relaxes.... feel the muscles in your neck and shoulders drifting down with gravity.... and relaxing even more deeply....

A more prolonged form of this breathing exercise is meditation. Some of you may not wish to meditate; just the feeling of being alone with yourself may create some anxiety. So begin with just a minute or two and add time as your comfort level grows.

Meditation

Meditation is easy to learn. The most difficult part may be finding the time. However, creating the time, whether it be every day or three times a week, can be tremendously rewarding, offering you relaxation, tranquility and even growth and insight. Remember that there is no one way to meditate. Often, the biggest obstacle is our own self-judgment or our attitude that we are not really in a meditative state. But the mere fact that you have taken out five or ten minutes to lie down or sit down quietly and breathe means that meditation is going on. Don't compare yourself to others and their meditation style. Meditation is a private affair. Above all, don't think you have failed if you do not continue it or if you think you are getting nothing from it. As you practice it more and more, you will feel that your body quiets down more easily and is more receptive to the messages that it receives.

Before meditation, go to a room where you won't be interrupted. Take the telephone off the hook or put the answering machine on. Sit in a comfortable chair or lie down on a carpet with a small pillow under your head if this feels comfortable to you. If you are in a seated position, I would recommend that you sit next to a glass of water. Sometimes it is good to have a ritual before you meditate. Placing a glass of water near you will help to set the tone to sit down or lie down quietly. Remember that in the beginning, your body may find five different reasons to get up and do something. You may feel fidgety or you may remember that you need to call someone. Ignore these inner promptings. Now is the time to just relax. Close your eyes.

Start by taking four slow breaths in and out through your nostrils. Now tell yourself to relax. Continue to breathe slowly in and out either in through the nose and out through the mouth or in and out through the nose, which ever is more comfortable. As you breathe, put your attention into your body. If you are having trouble relaxing, tell each part of your body to relax. Simply say, "my head is relaxed, my eyes are relaxed, my legs are relaxed, my heart is relaxed and calm," etc. At this time, many thoughts may run through your consciousness. Do not resist them, but don't focus on them either. Merely note them and let them pass. If the thoughts continue to come, imagine opening a door and saying to all those thoughts, "I know you are there, but I don't want to let you in." Actually see or feel these thoughts going out the door and close the door behind them. You may need to do this a few times.

When you are relaxed enough, you will begin breathing naturally. Take in more slow deep breaths every so often and remember to let the air out slowly. When you are relaxed, imagine that you have an inner physician, healer or very wise spiritual leader within you. This inner healer is very wise and loving and may be called upon for any number of ideas, knowledge or guidance. Tell this healer or spiritual being about your pain, particularly about your heart. Let yourself flow with this process. See what you need to express to this inner wise healer and then ask for help or guidance. Perhaps you want to attract a perfect support system. Know that you have a right to ask for this. You can even ask for healing. Do not be afraid. And when you ask for help, you may have feelings come up. If you feel sadness, for example, let yourself cry. Whatever you feel, just allow it to come out completely. Try to stay open to receive insights, but don't struggle with it.

Just trust that this guidance will come in various ways. Many patients tell me that after they performed a meditation, an insight came to them at a later time. You might feel some inspiration to call someone, perhaps a relative or friend. Follow whatever instincts you have. When the experience feels complete, take a few more breaths in and out and thank the wise healer or spiritual being for the message. Take a few more deep breaths and now slowly open your eyes.

You can use meditation for relaxation and also to "reframe" your heart disease, looking at it from a different perspective. Through meditation some of my patients have gained tremendous insight into their emotional and spiritual beings. Some of them have received the message that their heart disease was really a gift to them, offering a new opportunity to experience life, relationships and whatever is most dear to their hearts. Meditation may also be an opportunity to help you work on some of your feelings, especially sadness and fear.

When you meditate, try not to intellectualize. Do not ask, for example, "why am I sad, or why am I angry or why am I so fearful?" Just experience the feeling. By doing this, you will be acknowledging your body and living in it. When you do this, you cannot live in denial. By experiencing your feelings, you can heal your body both emotionally and physically. Remember that repetition is very important in visualizing yourself as feeling healthier, stronger and filled with vitality. Working through your mind's eye in this way will certainly help to heal your body and your heart.

If you feel connected to meditation and wish to take this to another level, I recommend trying mental imaging, a way to heal your heart using your own imagination.

Mental Imaging:
Healing Your Heart with Your Imagination

Have you ever wondered why books about spiritual quests and dramatic recoveries from disease are perennially on the best-seller lists? I think it's because we all want to know how we can harness our inner resources to affect the important things in our lives. Your imagination is one of those inner resources and it can have a profound effect upon your health. Taking full advantage of your imagination can help you recover from heart disease.

How can you turn your imagination into a tool for healing yourself? One avenue is through mental imaging, sometimes known as guided imagery or visualization. I use mental imaging with my patients and instruct them how to use it on their own. Over the past 10 years, more and more physicians are recommending the use of mental imaging for patients with serious illnesses such as heart disease and cancer. This is because research has shown that mental imaging works.

In mental imaging, you use your visual imagination to mobilize your inner natural healing power through your emotions. By accessing the right brain in mental imagery, fantasy or visualization, you can imagine you are experiencing something and your body reacts as if it's actually happening. For instance, if you create a strong mental image of cutting into a bright yellow, aromatic, sour lemon, you may have a strong physical response such as a tensing of your facial muscles and lips as your mouth begins to water. Stop reading and try it; it really works. You're using mental imagery to elicit a specific physiological response. Your mind speaks to your body and your body speaks back to your mind. You can learn to use this mind/body dialogue to heal your heart.

Remember, like all emotions, the powerful images and feelings evoked by mental imagery can create physiological changes in the body which can affect the functioning of the heart and other organs. But the physiological aspects of emotions can also heal the heart. The goal of mental imagery is to use the imagination to elicit those emotions so that their physical expression can heal the heart.

For some of you, these ideas may sound like "New Age" mumbo jumbo. But I can assure you that imagery is an adjunct to traditional medical treatment that works. The relationship between mental imagery, relaxation, physiological responses and behavior has been documented in many scientific studies. For example, a technique called relaxation with guided imaging (RGI) has been shown to decrease anxiety, reduce stress and depression, increase feelings of well-being and influence the outcome of serious illness. In one study on RGI and its effect on the immune system, subjects had significantly lower symptoms of rapid heartbeat, breathing difficulties and jaw clenching after using RGI. In other studies, cancer patients taught various mental imaging techniques used them to successfully enhance the effectiveness of radiation and chemotherapy.

A Healing Journey

Let's try a mental imaging exercise to put you in touch with your heart and body on both a physical and spiritual level. Just remember that there is no one right way to do this; the important thing is to allow the imagery to bring out your feelings. Then follow those feelings. If you do not experience an image or emotional response to your first few attempts, don't become discouraged. Journeying inward is a process that often develops slowly over time. This exercise may work best for you if you tape it yourself and then play it back or have a friend record it for you. You can also ask a friend to take you through the process by reading this exercise to you.

Before you start, follow my instructions for meditation, but instead of sitting, recline or lie down on the floor. Make yourself comfortable. Close your eyes and take a few deep breaths through your nostrils. Take a moment to feel how wonderful it is to have the floor support your back, buttocks and legs. Feel the breath going in and out. Do this for a minute or two until you're totally focused on your rhythmic breathing.

As soon as you're comfortable, try to visualize your heart. What does it look like as it beats steadily in your chest? Next, I want you to see your heart as a living pump pushing its life-sustaining force throughout your body. Hear the gentle pulsations of your heartbeat. Make a mental picture of this, looking at how each and every one of your cells is being bathed in this life-sustaining force. Once you begin to feel the strength of your heart beating, give your heart a color. Visualize it as whatever color first leaps to mind. Ask yourself how much space this color occupies in your chest. Does it fill your chest? Or is it just a small colored area inside your heart? Does the color radiate outward to fill your body? Does the color extend beyond the limits of your body? Can you see this color glowing all around you? I want you to exhale your breath into it, fill it with your breath and feel its presence.

Now, as you see this color inside your chest, give the color a voice. What is it saying to you? Is it a joyful voice? Does it sing? Or is it a sad voice? Do you hear your heart weeping?

Is the voice a shout of outrage or anger? Or is it a groan of despair or even a cry? Or do you only hear silence, does your heart have no voice or is it simply not speaking right now?

What is the voice of your heart saying? What is it trying to express? If you can't hear this clearly at first, then ask the color inside your chest for these answers and listen for its message. It may be very simple, only one word, or a moan or cry. After you've received your message, tell it to your heart. See your heart's color, hear its voice and tell your heart that it is healing. Then tell yourself that you are healing your heart, that you are nurturing your heart—and with it, your life.

Now, let all your mental images fade. Open your eyes slowly and again feel the presence of the floor against your back. Lie on the floor quietly until you feel you want to get up.

Some will get a lot from this exercise and some may get little or nothing. Either is okay; this exercise is not about performance. It is about getting in touch with your heart on a body level. If you didn't get anything this time, don't worry. Try to repeat it every day and eventually you will get results. The investment is only five to ten minutes of your time each day.

If you do get something from the exercise, listen to the message. If you feel sadness or if you begin to cry, you'll know that your heart is sad. That's fine, because this is intended to bring you awareness and to help you get you in touch with your feelings. If strong sadness or other uncomfortable feelings come up, I urge you to talk about them with a social worker, a therapist, a nurse, your doctor, your clergyman or a friend. Remember: when you talk about your feelings and share yourself with others, it sets the stage for healing. It is also crucial for you to feel your emotions as well. Consider crying—a magical heart-healer.

Crying

Crying, next to love, is perhaps the most healing activity for the heart. Crying frees the heart of muscular tension and rigidity. Sobbing also enhances oxygen delivery. Man is the only primate able to weep for emotional reasons. Why are tears so copious during emotion? Tennyson wrote:

"Home they brought her warrior dead.
She nor swoon'd nor utter'd cry;
All her maidens watching, said, "She must weep or she will die . . ."

Tennyson knew the value of weeping as nature's way to release the pain of heartbreak and prevent death. Crying is also necessary so heartbreak will not lead to heart disease. Any expression of feeling will help to heal your heart. Despite what we are taught, it is not weak to show your feelings. In fact, it is far healthier than "stuffing" your feeling and seething silently.

How can you handle your most powerful emotions? One of the best ways is to cry. In my workshops on healing the heart, I have generally found that men and women who don't cry tend to get heart disease.

As a cardiologist and psychotherapist, I knew how valuable it was to cry, but for years in my own private therapy, I found crying almost impossible. I knew I was coronary-prone and that I had a very tight chest. I began to search for the answers in my own therapy. Why was it so difficult for me to cry? Perhaps, holding back my tears helped me to survive as a child. Not crying was a way of holding back from my parents.

Moreover, I never saw my own father cry. On a conscious level, I probably felt it was not "manly" to cry. Although I greatly reduced the tension in my chest through therapy, I still could not get into deep feelings or crying. Therapy had opened the door to my sadness, but it took a real life experience to open my heart and finally experience crying.

In an earlier chapter I discussed how healing it had been for me to experience deep sobbing with both the death of my father and the heartbreak of my medical malpractice suit. These life experiences coupled with psychotherapy (which had given me permission to cry) were absolutely essential in assisting me to experience deep levels of sadness. The ability to feel emotions deeply, to cry during times of intense sadness and heartbreak are, I believe, essential in the prevention of heart disease. Many times in my office when I see other men and their inability to cry, I make it a point to touch their sadness in an attempt to open a door in their healing process.

A good cry literally lightens your heart. I emphasize that this is not just an image, but a *medical fact*. Research has shown that tears emitted during emotional crying differ physiologically from those provoked by irritants. Based on my training as a bioenergetic therapist, I believe strongly that crying opens the chest, allowing the energy bound by stress to be released from the thoracic cavity. Sobbing enhances healthy breathing at the same time that it discharges sadness and anger from your body.

Crying is our earliest expression, the first reaction we have as we exit the womb. Crying, the body's basic primitive release mechanism, is absolutely essential in opening the heart. It is better, however, not to cry alone, especially if loss, isolation or alienation are at the root of your reason for sadness.

If possible, do your crying with a "witness," a friend, loved one or concerned therapist. Such a person can not only help you keep the process going, but can offer understanding, comfort and unconditional support as you access your heartbreak. Research has also shown that crying actually cleanses the eyes and produces chemicals in your body that cause your cells to relax. That's why you often feel so relieved after a good cry. While crying is one of the most powerful ways to release emotional energy, any wholehearted physical expression of feeling will have a positive benefit.

At this point, I'm sure that many of you are thinking: "It's hard for me to express myself through crying. What shall I do?" I suggest going to the movies or renting some videos. *Dr. Zhivago* has always been a tear-jerker for me. The movies *Rudy* and *Hoosiers* also make me cry every time I watch them. Many of us are unable to cry for ourselves; we may view our sadness as self-pity, dismissing our tears before they can develop. But, through empathizing with others in heartbreaking situations, we may give ourselves permission to cry. A movie may be a safe catalyst for the deep sadness to begin to emerge that is buried within you.

If a movie does cause your eyes to water, just go with the flow and try to get into a deeper expression of crying. If you can cry and sob from your belly and diaphragm, you will be experiencing the most healing involuntary emotion you can access. Movies can also be a recipe for laughter. Laughter, like crying, is also a tremendous remedy for the heart.

Laughing

Laughter is a medicine with no equal. When you laugh fully, breathing increases, freeing up the rigidity in the chest, diaphragm and even deep down into the psoas muscles. Laughing is a way to experience strong feeling just as crying is. In fact, strenuous laughter often turns into tears. I have frequently seen my patients in group situations get so carried away with their laughter that they begin to cry.

I have also seen many patients laugh as a way of denying or blocking their sadness. For them laughing is acceptable, but crying is not. I experienced this on a recent fishing trip with five of my friends in New Brunswick, Canada. One of those friends, a patient, was also a Vietnam combat veteran. He told me how very difficult it was for him to cry or experience anger. I believe that he shut down many of his feelings to protect himself from his emotions during his tragic combat experiences in Vietnam. This ability to "disconnect" from his emotions may have been essential to his survival during the war. But that which may save us at one point in our lives may set a pattern that can hurt us later on.

This friend does, however, enjoy laughing. In fact, his laugh has such an uncontrollable quality that it is contagious. When he laughs, others in the room pick up on his energy and laugh uncontrollably right along with him. This happened throughout our trip. All of us laughed along with him all week, nicknaming him the "laughing hyena." Laughing is a good way to connect with other people if you feel emotionally shut down. Laughing not only heals one emotionally, but physically as well.

Norman Cousins was one of the first to encourage laughter and identified it as the most powerful healing remedy for his severe collagen and arthritic conditions.

According to one of my teachers, Alexander Lowen, spontaneous uncontrolled laughing creates convulsive reactions in which the voice and breathing are charged and mobilized. A release of tension results from the convulsive movements of the body. According to Lowen, laughter ends with an upward turn of the face in opposition to crying which turns the face downward.

I recall a therapy session I had with Lowen several years ago. As I was performing breathing exercises to open up the energy of the chest, I felt rather silly and slowly started to laugh. Lowen instinctively and intuitively knew that this would facilitate the opening up of the rigidity in my chest. As I laughed, he started to tickle me, encouraging me to laugh uncontrollably. I remember feeling really good after that session because I had had the experience of being totally out of my head and into my body.

I experienced a similar mind/body situation on a rough ferry boat ride from Newfoundland to Nova Scotia a few years ago. There was a horrible storm. I remember the water breaking over the deck, six stories high. Many people started to get fearful. Many became seasick. I was afraid that I would also become ill. Fortunately, there was an old comedy movie on board called *The Pink Panther*. I took a chance and watched it. The result was that I laughed so hard that I was too preoccupied to become seasick. Laughing at this slapstick comedy made me feel silly and childlike. While about 90 percent of the passengers on the boat were sick, laughing had literally saved me by distracting me from the rough voyage as well as from my fear of seasickness and loss of control.

Laughter as a spontaneous release of energy has the potential to be extremely therapeutic in releasing trapped energy within the chest. Although it is not always easy to see the lighter side of things, if you can find some humor in most situations, you will begin to lighten up. I believe too many of us avoid humor and laughter. As a physician I see this a lot among my own colleagues. Most of the time, we physicians are just too serious. We need to remember how important it is not to stifle the impulse to laugh.

If you have heart disease—or even if you don't, try being more silly and uninhibited. Rent some comedy videos such as *The Pink Panther* or some of the old Laurel and Hardy movies that are guaranteed to provoke spontaneous laughter. Laughing, like crying and any other spontaneous release of energy promotes respiration, thus providing the heart with much needed oxygen. Laughter also frees up the tensions that are locked inside the chest cavity. Laughter is one of several spontaneous emotional releases that are essential to support the health of the heart.

Sexuality

Getting in touch with your negativity, learning about your dark side, expressing anger, experiencing crying and taking in love and intimacy are all ways to mobilize the energies that ultimately can heal the heart. But what about sex? Is there a connection between sexual satisfaction on both physical and emotional levels and heart disease? Before we embark on a discussion of sexuality and how it relates to the heart, it is necessary to briefly discuss the psychoanalytic therapy originating from the works of Wilhelm Reich.

Reich, a psychiatrist and student of Freud, proposed that healthy sexuality could cure all the ills of mankind. This belief is also reflected in ancient Chinese Taoist texts and practices. Reich was known for his writings on the relationship of disease, emotions and the denial or absence of sexual pleasure. In his renowned book, *The Function of the Orgasm*, Reich states:

> Psychic health depends upon orgastic potency, upon the degree to which one can surrender to and experience a climax of excitation in the natural sex act. It is founded upon the healthy

character attitude of the individual's capacity for love. Psychic illnesses are the result of the disturbance of the natural ability to love. In the case of orgastic impotence, from which the overwhelming majority of people suffer, damming up of biological energy occurs and becomes the source of irrational actions. The essential requirement to cure psychic disturbances is the reestablishment of the natural capacity for love. It is dependent upon social as well as psychic conditions.

Thus, Reich believed that psychic illnesses were the consequence of sexual disturbances both for the individual as well as for the culture. He also believed that people who were brought up with a negative attitude regarding life and sexuality developed chronic muscular spasms and anxieties.

Reich understood that the sexual experience was an expansive process of biological pleasure which was tremendously healing, not only to the psychological and emotional aspects of the individual, but the physical aspects as well. He also believed in the correlation between one's overall body energy and sexual energy. Sexuality was seen as one way of releasing the blocked energetic charges contained within the body.

Building on Reich's theory, Alexander Lowen developed his own therapy techniques. As a student of Reich's, Lowen also believed that repressed emotions, especially unresolved sexual conflicts, can affect the way we breathe. The blocked energy flow in respiration can also affect the heart over time through the armoring and rigidification processes that occur in the chest wall, diaphragm and pelvis. Lowen believes that counseling, breathing techniques and the release of buried emotions as well as the expression of healthy sexuality are all conducive to healing the heart.

Several years ago, I conducted a Heart/Health Workshop with Lowen. Approximately 20 of my patients with heart disease attended an afternoon workshop regarding sexuality. The group consisted of both men and women. Lowen worked with every one of these patients on deep core issues regarding love, intimacy and sexuality. The common thread these cardiac participants discovered through this process was an unsatisfactory sex life. Though only some of the participants focused on issues of impotence, frigidity and lack of orgastic potency, all participants indicated a lack of physical and emotional satisfaction in intimacy with their partners. Although this was only a small workshop of 20 people, the findings were similar to reports in the medical literature.

For example, some studies suggest that a failure to reach orgasm may have a negative impact on the heart. One investigation surveyed 200 hospitalized women. The control group of 100 women with varied diagnoses was compared with the study group of 100 women with heart attacks. In the 100 women hospitalized for other illnesses, a 24-percent incidence of dissatisfaction with sex was reported. In the heart attack group, however, participants reported a 65-percent occurrence of frigidity and dissatisfaction with the sexual act. Similar findings were noted in men. A similar study of male sexual dysfunction was conducted with 131 men aged 31 to 86 who had been hospitalized for heart attack. Approximately two-thirds of the men in this investigation reported experiencing significant problems with their sexuality for weeks or months prior to heart attack. These studies, when added to the small unpublished data gathered from our own workshop, suggest a relationship between sexual dysfunction and coronary heart disease.

How are sexuality and the heart connected? As a cardiologist and psychotherapist I have often pondered this question. Although sexuality can have different connotations with respect to love, intimacy and physical expression, the fact remains that sexual satisfaction is highly conducive to the health of the heart. This is hardly surprising when you consider that unsatisfying sexual relationships often lead to feelings of failure, worthlessness, isolation, alienation and loss of control.

Such feelings can easily lead to self-protective, intimacy-avoiding behaviors. These behaviors may successfully shield the individual, protecting him or her from further disappointing or humiliating experiences, while also deepening the sense of isolation and alienation.

Desperate attempts to compensate by exerting control in areas of life outside the sexual arena may result in rigid behaviors and strategies that actually repel other people. This scenario all too often ends in a downward-circling spiral carrying the individual deeper into depression and resentment, leading to a diminished ability to find joy and meaning in life. A serious, literal heart "break" occurs as emotional and social stressors come together with a devastating impact on the health of the heart.

Studies have shown that the most physically and emotionally satisfied sexual partners were married couples. According to the authors of the book, *Sex in America,* married women reported a much higher frequency of orgasm than women who were unmarried. The authors also indicated that happiness with a sexual partner appeared to be correlated with happiness in life.

Following extensive interviews, subjects who described themselves as happy in general also reported being happy with their sex lives. It was also interesting to note that those with higher levels of self-esteem and happiness reported more frequent sexual activity. Although this study did not comment on longevity of life, there have been studies demonstrating that a healthy sexual life within a committed relationship can be correlated with longevity.

Have you ever wondered why some elderly people look much younger than their stated age while some younger people look so much older? This observation was studied by a Russian gerontologist who examined 15,000 individuals over the age of 80 in provinces of the former Soviet Union. He found four common denominators or markers for longevity.

People who lived the longest reported working out-of-doors, high levels of physical activity and a diet of grains, fresh fruits and vegetables. But two of the four common denominators involved relationship, intimacy and sexuality.

The author indicated that many of these individuals continued to have an active sex life well into theirs 80s and 90s. Aging couples who are committed to one another's pleasure and sexually open can adapt sexually to the aging process. Although longevity and sexuality appear to be connected in these population studies, we have yet to explain why healthy sexuality is so supportive and nurturing to the heart.

Sexuality includes both emotional and physical expressions. On an emotional level, sexuality provides a sense of security, connectedness and emotional intimacy. When sexuality is an expression of love, the energies of the partners can fuse in harmony like two tuning forks vibrating with the same frequency. Feelings of warmth, connectedness and emotional intimacy can help open our hearts. Ask any woman or man who has experienced a deep emotional feeling in sexuality and they will tell you how vulnerable they feel. When sexuality is experienced on a heart level, the partners feel fulfilled. However, when sex is performed solely for the ego, the heart is not involved on an emotional level. The heart and genitals fail to connect. When the heart is left out of the sexual act it becomes isolated, uninvolved and cold. When the heart and the pelvis are not connected, a splitting is created in the flow of the body's energies. Orgasm in such a context is incomplete.

However, if the heart and the pelvis are connected on both emotional and physical levels, the spontaneous release that occurs creates a discharge of energy resulting in profound parasympathetic activation and expansion of the body's vitality. This expansion or opening is truly healing for the heart.

According to Reich, the complete orgasm response involves the entire body. The spontaneous release resulting from orgasm creates tremendously pleasurable convulsions, pelvic thrusts and body waves. Such an involvement literally overwhelms the ego, surrendering the self out of head and into the body. Full-bodied sensation with pleasurable energy streamings creates a deep and profound sense of connectedness and satisfaction that is truly experienced by the heart. Following such an emotional and physical release, lovers frequently collapse, falling asleep and waking up several hours later feeling truly connected, joyful and alive.

Reich had a strong belief that the orgasm reflex was the most important entity in healing the body. He also believed that the orgasm reflex could be initiated by breathing techniques. Reich believed that neurotic people were incapable of breathing out deeply and evenly in one breath. He described this type of exhalation as fragmented, as the neurotic individual was quick to revert to inhalation. Reich reported this breathing pattern in one of his patients, metaphorically saying, "it is as if an ocean wave dashed against a rocky shore—it doesn't go any further."

The inhibition of breathing occurring in the abdomen and diaphragm causes a respiratory block that can be deleterious to the heart. Reich indicated that when a person breathes naturally and deeply, his head spontaneously moves back at the end of the breath. Reich believed that spontaneous breathing, like the orgasm reflex, could produce wave-like contractions in the abdomen, chest and pelvis. This involuntary activity arising out of the body has no attachment to the ego. Such a release of energy connotates the attitude of "sexual" surrender. It is this spontaneous release of energy, whether occurring in breathing, laughing, crying or sexual expression, that is so nurturing to the pulsatory actions of the heart. The satisfaction in sexuality does not only occur from voluntary pleasurable movements but also from the involuntary ones.

It is the uncontrollable, involuntary movement inducing physical surrender that is a sign that the ego has been set aside and "life" has taken over. On a deep level, the inability to surrender is a core issue of many cardiac patients. Being able to surrender is a hallmark of cardiac health. This is where women have a health advantage over men.

Women are truly the stronger sex in this regard. The ability to surrender is more highly developed in women than in men. Why is this so? The answer, perhaps, is rooted in the cyclic nature of a woman's biology, which requires her to accept monthly physical and psychoemotional changes which involve the buildup and discharge of energy throughout her childbearing years. Women must surrender to the emotional and physical sensations of menstruation. I believe one of the reasons that premenopausal women have far less heart disease than men, aside from the cardio-protective effects of their high estrogen levels, is the natural protective mechanism of menstruation. Menstruation is a way of releasing energy in the body.

Unfortunately, because of their different physiology, men's nature seems to be more linear, more goal-oriented and less inclined to submit to the demands of nature. Just like Engel who was able to save his heart through understanding the root cause of his bleeding hemorrhoids, many women "save their hearts" through the release that comes with menstruation. Although many women don't realize it, this emotional and physical release of tensions is extremely healing to their hearts.

Women are also naturally able to release energy in their bodies through breast-feeding and childbirth. When a woman puts her whole heart into the endeavor of delivering a baby, it is a majestic act for healing the heart. Such an experience creates a tremendous surge of energy to the pelvis, allowing the dissipation of tension in the body which is then replaced by joy. I have also heard women comment that a great energy pulses through them during childbirth, a sense of something powerful and immense overtaking them. When the ego is overwhelmed by such physical and emotional sensations, the body takes over. When natural pulsatory mechanisms prevail, the heart is soft and unopposed. A feeling of unity is established throughout the body.

Perhaps Reich was right when he stated that true orgastic potency could be identified as cosmic revelation. The forces of love and sexuality, like birth, death and other all-consuming experiences demanding our unconditional surrender, can create a state of sacred fusion and a sense of union deep within the core of our hearts on both metaphorical and physical levels. Such forces are truly cosmic, as the pulsations in our human bodies reflect the pulsation of the cosmos in the heavenly bodies. When such energy is realized in the heart or in the core of our being, our life force pulsates and radiates like a twinkling jewel.

Nutritional Healing

Throughout the course of this book, I have been discussing the concept of energy and how it relates to illness. In reality, the most important factor in determining health and illness is how much energy an individual has and how that energy is utilized by the body. The generation of energy includes two components. The first involves maintenance of adequate oxygen levels through a healthy pattern of breathing. The second component involves the intake of essential nutrients required for the production of high-energy ATP-ADP bonds required to drive the machinery of the cell. Homeostasis requires an appropriate balance of oxygen and nutritional components such as enzymes, co-factors, vitamins and minerals that allow cells to function with ease. Any major disruption may precipitate *dis-ease*. Thus, the concept of energy is both quantitative and qualitative.

Unfortunately, many of us are deficient in such natural nutrients as magnesium, coenzyme Q_{10}, B-vitamins, flavonoids, carotenoids, and so on. A deficiency in any of these components will impair the healthy functioning of our metabolism. Such a deficiency, often undetected or unsuspected, contributes year after year to the impaired functioning of our cells and bodies. Consider, for example, the treatment of depression. We all know how valuable cognitive and body-oriented psychotherapy are in mobilizing both insight and energy. However, many cases of depression require additional neurotransmitters frequently facilitated by psychotropic medicines. Moreover, up to 70 percent of cases are deficient in the mineral magnesium. Therefore, without cellular biochemical support, psychotherapy alone would be inadequate in treating the whole person. The same is true for the heart.

The heart requires tremendous biochemical support. We know that the contractive ability of the heart depends on the functional capacity of myocardial cells to expand and contract. This is pulsation. However, in the defective pulsation of congestive heart failure, there are insufficient myocardial contractive forces. Heart failure is literally an energy-starved heart. In order to treat the heart appropriately, the cardiologist must consider the molecular and cellular components of the heart, the biochemistry of "pulsation." Consider the miracle nutrient coenzyme Q_{10}. Q_{10} is a vital nutrient found naturally in sardines, salmon, mackerel and beef heart. As a powerful antioxidant and membrane stabilizer, coenzyme Q_{10} prevents the depletion of substances which recharge the energy system in the body cells. This energy system is critical for anyone with heart muscle disease. As the heart muscle continually uses oxygen and consumes huge amounts of energy, heart muscle cells can greatly benefit from the energy boost of coenzyme Q_{10}. In fact, the amount of coenzyme Q_{10} is naturally 10 times higher in the heart than any other organ.

This is why coenzyme Q_{10} has proven to be life-saving for patients with congestive heart failure. Since cardiac muscle is one of the few tissues in the body to be continuously aerobic, a constant supply of energy is required. Q_{10} enhances ATP-ADP production in the mitochondria, thus enhancing intrinsic energy to the cell.

The heart is extremely vulnerable to nutritional deficiencies. Since the heart is the most susceptible of all the organs to premature aging and free radical invasion, clinical research has clearly documented the heart's receptivity to the benefits of targeted nutrients, phytonutrients, antioxidants and other nutritionals.

Scientific evidence has demonstrated over and over again that diet modification, antioxidant vitamins and minerals as well as other nutritionals can protect us against heart disease. Phytonutrients such as natural flavonoids and carotenoids found in fresh fruits and vegetables and vitamins C, E and beta carotene have powerful antioxidant effects which are protective to the heart. In addition, minerals like selenium and nutrients such as coenzyme Q_{10} will minimize free radical risk, stabilize membranes and help prevent the presence of oxidative stress on the cardiovascular system. The B complex vitamins particularly folic acid, B_{12} and B_6 are also essential in the prevention of premature coronary artery disease. These nutrients combat the deleterious effects that blood homocysteine has on our blood vessels.

A healthy diet supplemented with antioxidants and phytonutrients is essential in the prevention and promotion of optimum cardiovascular health. There are also a number of herbs, botanicals, amino acids, essential fatty acids and other nutrients that are nurturing to the heart, including garlic and onions. It is beyond the scope of this book to include an in-depth discussion of nutritional healing for the heart. This subject is vast, all-encompassing and merits a full discussion on its own.

My previous book, *Optimum Health*, contains a comprehensive discussion of how antioxidants and other nutritional strategies may be used to nurture and heal the heart. For other valuable books on this subject, refer to my list of recommended books on page 249.

Touch Therapy

Animals can teach us a lot about human contact. Have you ever noticed how a dog or a cat will nuzzle up close to you and want to be touched or petted? Have you ever experienced a dog left alone all day who showers you with love and demands your attention when you return home? Such a pet would rather be touched than fed.

Canine studies have shown that the mere presence of a human being will increase heart rate, systolic blood pressure and coronary blood flow. However, when the dog is petted, the whole process is reversed, dropping the heart rate to below the baseline. Petting a dog has also been shown to reverse the conditioned response to an electric shock. When shocks are given to dogs in experimental settings, the usual response is an acceleration in heart rate, which is a response to pain and fear. However, the same dogs showed a paradoxical decrease in heart rate when they were petted during the shock, indicating that petting overrode the pain and fear responses of the heart. Thus, touch therapy is very stabilizing.

In humans, too, touch therapy or massage appears to be associated with a decreased heart rate, decreased blood pressure and increased endorphin release resulting in an increased sense of relaxation and heightened well-being. In humans, massage can be considered a nonchemical tranquilizer with absolutely no side effects. The parasympathetic activation of massage provides a healing balance to the typical sympathetic overdrive of the coronary prone person. The effects of massage can be an integral component in healing the heart. In this situation, the bodywork technique (i.e. massage) places the client in a passive condition in which he or she is a recipient of the therapeutic touch of the health care provider. This is in direct contrast to body-oriented psychotherapies where the client is an active participant in the body exercise.

There are many types of bodywork that are nurturing to

the heart and body, "different strokes for different folks." Not every form of body work appeals to every person. People have different body types, different medical problems, different emotional histories and different needs. Luckily, there are many forms of bodywork currently available to choose from and most patients are able to find a method that works for them.

For my own growth and development over the past two decades, I have personally experienced many body therapies. For example, I have experienced the controlled precision of Shiatsu (accupressure massage). I have also been exposed to Trager massage, which includes rocking the body and its limbs. Then there is the more familiar Swedish massage which includes stroking, kneading, pressure, friction, percussion and vibration of the musculoskeletal body structure. I also recommend rolfing, a very vigorous method which breaks up myofascial adhesions and helps to realign the posture and refigure the body. Psychotherapist Fritz Perls credited rolfing with saving his life after a heart attack.

Although there are many different types of bodywork available, they all have a common thread: nurturance through touch. The core message of massage lies in its unique way of communicating without words. When receiving a good massage, a person usually falls into a mental-physical reverie. The person is not asleep, but neither is he or she fully awake. Massage facilitates this altered state, which is especially beneficial to the heart of the Type-A coronary-prone individual. Receiving therapeutic touch in an altered state can help the alienated Type A client reconnect to others as well as to him or herself. This in itself is a crucial step in healing.

The benefits of massage are legion. Physically, it can tame the fight-flight response, decreasing heart rate and blood pressure. In addition, massage, Trager, rolfing and other forms of bodywork can also facilitate emotional release. Memory is deeply buried within our musculature. Bodywork can access old traumas, release stored emotional charges and free up the body's energy previously locked in chronic, defensive holding patterns. For example, the release of sadness often occurs as a result of body manipulation. A good massage therapist will encourage this emotional release while providing a safe space for its expression. Once freed up, these energies and emotions can be redirected toward healing.

Touch is the most essential and ubiquitous sense we have. It is the first to be perceived by the newborn. It is often the last to leave us. The familiar phrase "losing touch" refers to a condition in which the individual, his perceptions of his environment and his relationship to that environment become "unreal." When we are able to take in nurturing touch in a therapeutic nonsexual context, this creates a deep connection to the self. Unfortunately, this connection is lacking in many of the Type-A, coronary-prone individuals that I treat. A major benefit of bodywork is to establish a reconnection to the self and others. This may occur in Swedish massage, Trager (a rocking type of massage) and to a greater degree in rolfing.

Rolfing entails intense and deep myofascial release. In rolfing, you must soften. You have no other choice. If you do not breathe into the resistance of the tissues being vigorously manipulated, you will experience some form of discomfort or pain. However, even this discomfort can be beneficial, since all feeling is healing. When we reach out and touch someone, we communicate on many levels. It is not cancer, heart disease or AIDS that represent the major disasters of the 20th century. It is man's alienation from man that is the common thread of unhappiness, discontent and disease.

Play

Play is one of the most healing things you can do for your heart health and your emotional well-being. Yet one of the most dismaying things I've learned in my years of medical practice is that adults no longer know how to play. In fact, when I ask my patients how they play, they often look at me with a blank expression on their faces.

Many of them answer that they "play" golf or tennis. But these are sports activities; they are not really play. One difference between sports and true play is that while I very seldom have heard of anyone dying while playing with their children or their dog or while tumbling around with their grandchildren, many of my patients have had heart attacks while "playing" golf, tennis or the most feared sport for sudden death, racquetball.

Although sports are enjoyable, they are not healing because they involve performance, competition and the need to win. Play is totally different. True play is spontaneous, has no set agenda, no rules or regulations and not even a desired outcome; when we play we are totally free. That is, we do things solely for joy and pleasure. When we play, we become totally absorbed in what we are doing; we are taken out of our heads and down into our bodies. Time stops for us.

Think of how completely absorbed five- or six-year-olds become when they are painting a picture. Within minutes, nothing else matters to them but the colors, the feel of the brush on the paper, the way the paint drips and blobs and runs, the way the colors mix and how closely they can match the picture with the image in their minds. Being carried away by their imagination and getting their inspirations down on paper is, for a short time, the single most important thing in the world to them. Everything else falls away—worries, fears, wants, needs, hunger—and is replaced by a sense of total involvement, excitement, satisfaction and gratification.

If you can play even partially this way, it completely cuts you free from stress and worry and helps heal your mind and heart. Because of this nearly miraculous benefit of play, I try to teach my patients to play like children. If, like most adults, they've forgotten how, I ask them to observe children and see what they do.

When you play like a child, you can experience a new sense of freedom. When you play with a child, let him take over and set the tone; if you take over, you'll lose all the spontaneity that goes along with playing with a child. Try swinging on a swing, blowing bubbles, finger-painting or playing catch. Children love to do these things. If you can lose yourself in these activities, you will find that you will love them too.

You can also play with your pets. Just get on the floor and roll around with your dog, or, if you have a cat, try rolling a ball, stalking the cat or tantalizing him with a piece of string. If you allow yourself to get carried away with this play, it will help you make contact with your animal and will also help you get in touch with the joy inside of you. This joy is your inner healing force.

Remember, play has no outcome, no goal. You need to play for play's sake alone and, when you play, try to bring out the little child inside you. Once you connect with your inner child (we all have one), it will bring you to another level of healing.

CHAPTER 8

—— ✧ ——

How It All Began

"Theoretically, I can imagine that someday we will regard our children, not as creatures to manipulate or change, but rather as messengers from a world we once deeply knew, but which we have long since forgotten, who can reveal to us more about the true secrets of life, and also about our own lives"

—ALICE MILLER,
For Your Own Good.

We have seen in earlier chapters that healing the heart involves a willingness on both conscious and unconscious levels to open one's heart to love. Although we cannot merely will our hearts to be loving, open and deeply connected, we can approach loving connections by becoming more vulnerable and by trying to reach out more toward others. Meditative states, deep crying, emotional release work and group process are experiential techniques that can get us in touch with ourselves. Even so, reopening the heart for an adult is often a slow, difficult process. For many of us, being truly open as children was a treacherous business. Melting the defenses we developed to survive in childhood requires a conscious awareness and integration of the events that caused us to armor ourselves as children.

It is the repressed experience of early childhood heartbreak that sets the stage for heart disease. In turn, the unconscious adult avoidance of intimacy arises as the result of the child's deep-seated fear to give and receive love wholeheartedly. It is this avoidance, leading to an inability to open the heart to loving connections, that creates the conflicts in our personalities that render us vulnerable to cardiac conditions. The love that we so desperately need may be the core vulnerability against which we have organized our very character structure.

But where does such love come from? Does it come from the mother or the father? Is love a learned experience? The answers to these questions are not simple. We do know that loving qualities, actions, energies and even words are transmitted to children from their parents. However, not all children are the recipients of these actions. Some are faced with cold, distant or distrustful parents. For them, the world may feel a bitter or emotionless place. Even for those who do receive more positive attentions, parental love can be confusing and even deforming if the love offered has narcissistic qualities, unconscious desires and other agendas attached to it.

The common thread in heartbreak for all of us, whatever the scenario, is that to a greater or lesser extent, parental needs were met at the expense of the developing child. To explore the roots of our unconscious fear of adult intimacy, it is necessary to journey back to earlier experiences of intimate relationships. Heartbreak can evolve from many sources: overinvolved, narcissistic parenting; distant, detached parenting; cold or cruel parenting; parents who were physically or emotionally unavailable. While this is an overly simplistic review of the psychological factors that may contribute to heartbreak, you may recognize small pieces of your own personal experiences in any of these categories.

In healthy parenting, the family unit is one in which the child is encouraged to explore who he or she is within safe and appropriate boundaries. Children are respected as unique individuals. They are guided and supported while mastering developmental tasks appropriate to their age. The self that is the child's is cherished and nurtured. Unconditional love and a positive regard for human nature are key ingredients in a healthy family unit.

Dysfunctional family relationships are essentially two polarities at opposite ends of the same continuum, with healthy family functioning in the center. One extreme is the distant, detached parent. Children may be left on their own to develop. Housing, food and shelter may be provided, but emotional attachments are loose to nonexistent. This emotional unavailability creates a family unit in which people live together, but have little direct involvement with one another's lives. Communication, comfort, contact, nurturing and guidance are foreign to these families. Children raised in these families have often learned to avoid contact or intimacy for fear of rejection and abandonment, laying down a characterological style that usually persists into adulthood. It is here that the child may develop the unconscious stance, "I don't need you anymore" or "I can do it myself" in order to survive the pain of detachment or abandonment. Or, the child may develop a clinging, dependent personality style due to persistently unmet needs for human love and caring.

In cold, cruel parenting, which is more prevalent than any of us would want to imagine, the child may be the victim of emotional or even physical and sexual abuse. The child's extension of self for contact may be met with indifference or even hatred and violence. The heartbreak is obvious for these individuals. Intimacy is a terrifying, painful experience, something to be avoided at all costs. Yet, even some individuals with this personal history will take repeated risks in the name of love, surviving repeated failures to find somewhere a safe connection. They, too, may be terrified to truly take in that which they so desperately seek.

Heartbreak is also experienced when the parental figure is physically unavailable. Even in the most healthy of families, a parent may go off to war, travel for a livelihood or even die. Separation from a loved parent, whether chronic, short-term or permanent, leads to profound heartbreak for the child, even if not totally conscious. Although a family member or step-parent may lovingly take the place of the lost love, the heart of the child will always remember the pain in some deep, sacred space.

Often more difficult to recognize is the overinvolved, en-meshed parent. To the outside world, it may look as if the parent were "perfect," caring and attentive in every way. But boundaries may become blurred; it may be very difficult to tease out the needs and wants of the child from those of the parent.

We have explored the difference between conditional and unconditional love in previous chapters. Conditional love car-ries with it double messages and narcissistic qualities; it is a love based on approval alone. Unconditional love, simply stated, means a love based on acceptance of an individual for who he or she is, not for what he or she does.

For example, if parental affection is expressed in direct pro-portion to how well-behaved the child is, the love is obviously conditioned on how well the child conforms. But what two-year-old is always well-behaved? Children have their mo-ments; they cry, they get angry, they soil their clothes, they have temper tantrums. At times they appear lazy, dirty and uncooperative; they argue and fight among themselves. They don't always fit our picture of what "good" children should be. Of course we all know that these characteristics are found in normal healthy children. However, when parents are con-vinced that they must teach their children how to behave in ways acceptable to themselves as adults, they require that the children act in a special way to fulfill parental needs.

Such needs can even go beyond behavior. Some parents need to control almost every aspect of their child's life. For example, if a school-age child wants to go to school wearing green, purple and orange and the parent is critical and interfering, a battle of wills may occur. The parent may believe that his or her image of being a "good parent" will be open to criticism if the child goes to school wearing an unconventional, brightly colored outfit. The parent has become overly invested in how the child acts and behaves. The child's actions are, to the narcissistic parent, not a statement of who the *child* is, but a mirror reflection of who the parent is. Thus, the parent's interference is based on their own image with an underlying fear of rejection by their own peers for allowing the child to dress in a nonconforming way. The parental investment is, therefore, personal at the expense of the child. Thus, parental narcissism interferes with the child's heartfelt desires and wishes. In actuality, if the child were to dress in a manner not acceptable to peers, negative comments by classmates would offer a quick solution to the mismatched wardrobe choices.

Children always tell the truth. Sometimes the truth is cold and cruel. Frequently the child on the other end of this experience will understand immediately. In other words, what may take a parent months of convincing can be accomplished by a peer group in a moment.

Children also need to be able to say "no" to their parents in a healthy way that establishes a firm boundary. If children are not allowed to say no to their parents, how are they going to have the confidence to say no to drugs and peer pressure?

At times, parental demands may be excessive, overbearing and overcontrolling. Forced submission in some children may create inner hostilities, as they receive the unspoken message that power and control are the entities that govern relationships. Usually, children will conform to parental wishes and restrict or inhibit their emotions. They will act in whatever way will fulfill parental desires. In this way, the "well-behaved" child will begin to live in a false self, not expressing his or her genuine feelings. When the well-behaved conforming child suppresses feelings to obtain love, the child is actually cheated emotionally. Children can only experience deep feelings safely if there is somebody there who accepts them fully, just the way they are.

Children who do not wish to risk losing vital parental love will learn to make adjustments and sacrifices. If young children grow up hearing familiar phrases like "Don't cry or I'll give you something to cry about" or "There's nothing to be afraid of," their bodies may freeze and contract in response to unremitting and overpowering parental demands. Alice Miller calls this "parental narcissism." Parents unknowingly, and the key word here is unknowingly, form and deform the lives of their children. It is a fact that parents have both the power and the control to influence the emotional lives of their children.

Of course, most of us as parents try to be caring and sensitive. We are full of good intentions and try to provide safe, nurturing environments. After all, parents are often right in their counsel and commands to their children. In most cases, they do know better. It is not our lack of knowledge that creates difficulty and problems, but our lack of *feeling* and our *insensitivity* to the child. Such blind, unconscious parental narcissism often causes us to fail to understand or even see the struggle and pain in our children.

Unfortunately, most parents are totally unaware of the damage that occurs. Most people who undergo some form of analysis or therapy later on in life enter with the belief that they grew up as happy, cheerful children. Early childhood experiences are frequently repressed, blocked and shut out, particularly if loss, abandonment, annihilation or fear is attached to them. It is only through therapy that early repressions are re-awakened. If parents are convinced that they must show their children how to be in the world, they take away independence, curiosity and creativity. Because parenting itself involves the unconscious acting out of unresolved issues from childhood, parents are not consciously aware of the projections of their own narcissistic wishes onto their children. Unconscious parental programming and a loss of sense of self may be the end result for the child.

According to Alice Miller and Alexander Lowen, in the majority of sensitive people, the true self remains deeply and thoroughly hidden. In *Prisoners of Childhood*, Dr. Miller states:

> How could you love someone you do not really know? How can you love something that has never been loved? So, it is that many a gifted person lives without any notion of his or her true self. Such people are enamored of an idealized, conforming false self. They will shun their hidden and lost true self, unless depression makes them aware of its loss or psychosis confronts them harshly with that true self, whom they now have to face and to whom they have been delivered up helplessly, as to a threatening stranger.

If young children suppress crying, anger and other emotions to avoid shame and humiliation, the denial of feeling occurs. If the child, from the very beginning, cannot experience true deep feelings, how can they ever love? The loss of the ability to take in love is, perhaps, the greatest risk factor for the heart. We shall see that unraveling this characterological issue is very important if we are to understand the emotional root of heart disease.

Although the connection between love and heart disease appears complicated we have seen over and over again that it does have profound merit. We have discussed love in terms of energy and expansive qualities and we know that love can be highly metaphoric. Some have tried to explain love through biochemistry in scientific terms. Others have defined love as a sense of being truly alive or as a cosmic force drawing one person to another. The poets tell us that the expression of love is the greatest feeling, with true romantic love being the "unreachable" star. But what actually is love? I have asked myself this question many times. We all know that love is a feeling, a genuine feeling that comes from the heart, but for many of us love can be just thoughts which Dr. James Lynch calls "narcissistic reverie." In a children's workshop many years ago I discovered the child's truth about love. Several children were my messengers in delivering their definition of love. Let me tell you about this workshop.

We placed twelve children, ages 7 to 13, in a group situation. We talked about life. We played. We discussed feelings and I tried to focus on what it was like to be a child. I remember how exhausted I was in that workshop. I had played a lot of soccer that day. Children have short attention spans and frequently we had to switch from play therapy to group talking. We took many breaks between the group therapy sessions. I found that children are a pleasure to work with. They tell the truth. They get right to the point. On this day, a group of several children revealed to me the true secrets of love.

They all said the same thing but in different words. It is very simple: children associate love with play. They revealed to me how good they felt when their parents played with them. They felt important and special. It also showed them that their parents loved them. Many growing children are, indeed, quite sensitive and shy and really do not understand the complexity of adult issues. Certainly, they cannot understand why adults are so preoccupied and so busy. Wanting to reach out, play and connect with their parents is the desire and even the need of every child. Children often feel rejected by the busy and hurried behavior of parents. Although this group of children did not say it in so many words, the withdrawal of play for them equaled the withdrawal of love. A 9-year-old told me, "My mom doesn't play with me anymore. She doesn't love me." A 10-year-old put it this way, "My dad is too busy, he doesn't come home at night. there must be something wrong with me."

Children often misinterpret parental withdrawal to mean that they are unlovable. On some deep level, the child will try repeatedly to connect with his parents. Eventually, the child may forfeit play for adult activity. He does what his parents do. He feels that in order to obtain love, he must be exactly like his parents. Frequently, such children will model the behavior of a parent and try to be "just like Dad." If they are in a household with two working parents or one over-worked parent, they may get the message that in order to be loved, they must work hard. Consciously, the child feels he is doing what his parents want. Unconsciously, it is here that the false connection between success and love takes root. The origin of Type-A behavior begins with the belief that success brings love. This distorted belief system can create worka-holic, narcissistic behaviors. If the child perceives that love is dependent upon what one does, such as high achievement and good grades rather than who one is, performance issues will predominate. If the child cannot perform up to standard, and most children feel ultimately that they do not, a basic insecu-rity develops. The result is often low self-esteem simmering just below the surface of competence and success.

Relatives, peer pressure and schools all contribute to rein-force this belief. Society places tremendous pressure on chil-dren to succeed. Children are encouraged to perform and excel at increasingly younger ages.

In addition, peer pressure and media influence push chil-dren to grow up fast socially, emotionally and even sexually. To add to the stress, these complex messages are often incon-sistent. Authority figures demand one kind of maturity while friends and the media demand another. Children become caught in the middle, probably not ready for either. Actually, what they really want and need is to be children a little longer.

Parental desires for achievement can inappropriately accel-erate childhood development. Parents frequently hurry children to act like adults by forcing major decisions upon them prematurely, pushing young children far beyond developmental abilities. This, once again, gives children the message "You are not acceptable the way you are." If children are being prodded to perform or entertain constantly, they are not left alone to experience the world at their own pace. In his provocative book, *The Hurried Child*, Dr. David Elkind offers many examples of how parents try to accelerate the developmental process of children, causing harmful psychological and physiological stress. Ignoring the fact that children are different from adults, children are clothed in tight designer jeans, prematurely accentuating their developing sexual characteristics. Parents tolerate a media environment that is explicitly sexual. Children are constantly being exposed to sexuality advertised in popular songs, television programming and the movies. Explicit adult sexuality and violence is too often available to children in their own homes through network programming and computers.

Other stress-making examples, according to Elkind, would include sending very young children to summer camps devoted to perfecting skills in computer use, competitive sports and the arts. This focus on skill acquisition, once again, drives home the message that childhood is not to be utilized in activities merely for fun. A preoccupation with organized sports may also usurp necessary playtime from children, resulting in less time to develop creativity and imagination. In this way, the left brain is developed in our society at the expense of the right brain.

Sometimes these efforts backfire. Research indicates that children pressured to learn to read prematurely usually derive less pleasure from reading later on in life. Those who have felt that acceptance by their parents depended upon higher achievement may be more susceptible to the appeals of cults, where one is initially accepted without any reservations or demands. Kids are rarely allowed to be "average." Those who don't perform at a high level often feel like failures. Although high-achieving behavior alone is not thought to contribute to coronary disease, such behavior associated with hostility, anxiety and time urgency are the hallmarks of the Type-A coronary-prone individual. Some children may become aggressive and achievement-oriented on their own, but aware parents can modulate this tendency by offsetting the urgent tempo with opportunities for play and relaxation.

In a world of high achievement, competition, child abuse, violent crime, global stress and emotional disruptions, many of our children live in continual fear and uncertainty. We must acknowledge that childhood suffering does go on and that it does not end with childhood. We need to be more respectful of our children's needs, feelings, creativity and individuality.

Of all the modern-day medicines, love is still the best remedy to assuage childhood pain and fear. But just as a lack of love or lack of play may result in false beliefs, the sudden loss of love can have serious consequences. Heartbreak is a universal consequence of human life. We have all experienced some heartbreak as very young children. The most serious and devastating heartbreaks, however, include the sudden withdrawal of love as a result of death or sudden abandonment. Let me tell you about Helen.

Helen was a woman in her late 40s seeking a cardiological evaluation for an arrhythmia. She was referred by her internist because of an abnormal electrocardiogram demonstrating several irregular heartbeats. She was scared to death about having heart disease. She could not even sleep at night in anticipation of the appointment she had made with me. In addition, she was suffering from hyperventilation, tingling in her arms and legs, shallow breathing, dizziness and sweating. These symptoms had intensified recently after she dropped her youngest daughter off at college. Experiencing loneliness and depression on such a deep level, she had begun to feel the pounding irregular sensations deep within the core of her body.

My first meeting with Helen was quite intriguing. As she discussed her cardiac sensations and irregular heartbeats, she was unaware of either heartbreak or fear. She was, however, in touch with her sadness. She acknowledged early childhood heartbreak, two marital failures and a recurrent theme of abandonment. As I spoke to Helen, I realized that she had suffered major heartbreak throughout her entire life.

Helen had suffered her first heartbreak at age three. At that time, she was abandoned by her father for no apparent reason. According to Helen, her father "just left the family" and was never seen again. For years, she experienced a deep longing for her father. In her 20s, she married and suffered a subsequent heartbreak when her husband left her at age 36. She remarried once again and divorced her second husband at age 46.

Having developed a strong distrust for men, Helen had avoided contact or intimacy in any relationship in the previous year. Although she could manage some sadness in private, she had difficulty crying. During this time of loneliness, there was considerable stress in her family life. Her middle daughter had a miscarriage and was involved in a bad marriage. Her oldest daughter was also getting divorced. This was a tremendous shock to Helen because she had believed her older daughter had a perfect marriage.

At the time of consultation, Helen was deeply sad and despondent. But perhaps the deepest sadness had occurred when she dropped her youngest daughter off at college. She had suddenly experienced panic and abandonment. It was at this time that her body had begun to fall apart. Helen had had a recent infection. She was also experiencing colitis and her heart was out of rhythm. When I told Helen that her cardiac arrhythmia was not the result of heart disease, but rather the result of acute heartbreak, she burst into tears. I explained to her that her issues of loneliness and abandonment were a core issue in her life. The recent empty nest with her youngest daughter going to college had provoked a reawakening of the abandonment she had experienced at age three.

During my evaluation with Helen, she openly broke into sobs. She too had the intuitive sense that she needed to love. But in order to love, she needed to trust. Although Helen was totally open to these remarks, she refused to become vulnerable and open her heart. She told me that she would rather let her body go and become overweight. She said, "Fat is unattractive and it will never get you hurt." Having been hurt by so many men, she had deliberately made herself sexually unattractive. By creating excessive padding as armoring, she felt that she was impenetrable. She had gradually developed the closed heart that had become her own trap. Helen was avoiding that which she wanted most in life.

On an unconscious level, Helen deeply needed a heart connection with a man. Suffering from heartbreak, Helen needed to work on issues of abandonment, longing and sadness as well as her anger and rage. Forgiveness is the antithesis to bitterness. Only through deep crying and sobbing and feeling the "wounded child" within her could Helen heal herself and, consequently, her heart.

Helen's case is not unusual. I have seen many patients with heart-related symptoms arising from childhood suffering. Abandonment at an early age may set the tone for acute heartbreak at a later stage, especially if the unconscious feelings of desertion are reawakened by recurrent experiences. Therefore, one acute heartbreak may set the stage for another and another until ultimately, the heartbreak is manifested in heart symptoms or even heart disease.

How can we heal our hearts? Throughout this book I have discussed the importance of crying, mental imagery, playing, laughing, breathing, emotional release and feelings of sexuality. Thus encouraging my patients to begin to feel and soften is a major step in their prevention of heart disease. It is essential for them to reframe their feelings and channel them in the direction of healing.

The trick here is to find the positive force in a negative event or experience, no matter how small; to laugh at yourself and not take everything quite so seriously; to communicate honestly and not internalize personal or work pressures; and to reach out and love, accepting in return the sincere affection of others. Keeping an open heart means being vulnerable and being able to forgive yourself and others over and over again. These are the positive forces and emotions that heal.

Since the path of our lives begins in our childhood, what can we do to enhance the self-love and self-esteem of our children? What can we do to reduce childhood fears and suffering in our own homes? The answers to these questions are not so simple. First of all, the child must feel loved and secure. We must remember that children follow what we do, not what we say. Children track our energy more than our words. As parents, it is important for us to identify and mobilize the positive forces in children that are not necessarily achievement oriented. As parents we need to slow down our own pace, thereby serving as helpful role models to our kids. If in their own lives, adults are relaxed and unhurried, children are less likely to develop consuming impatience and frustrations. As adults, we can counterbalance the constant peer competition among children. Wining need not always be paramount. Experiences gained and the effort expended are far more important than the destination or the goal. Fairy tales and creative stories can also enhance the process of developing self-awareness, encouraging and moving children away from the overstimulation that our high-tech, computerized society offers.

Children have the same basic fears, needs, securities and hopes as adults. They need to know that they are okay, that they are accepted for who they are and not for what their parents and teachers want them to be. They need to know that it is *all right* to fail. They need to know through our words and actions that they are loved. Children require our love, affection, patience and support. As we observe our children and share in their special moments, we can begin to appreciate their aliveness without interfering with their feelings, beliefs and attitudes.

We need to learn to accept our children as they are, as

unique individuals bringing their own special purpose to life. The gifts of love and acceptance are valuable gifts that each adult can give to the children in his or her life. And they are probably the best preventive medicine we have today. It is with these presents that we will begin to reduce childhood stress and assuage childhood suffering. It is then that we offer one of the best gifts of all: the gift of health. Children are, indeed, the messengers of our own past and they do reveal to us the true secrets of life. A re-experience of our own childhood is perhaps our most difficult task in our journey of healing the heart. One way to do this is to consider a group process experience, described in the chapter that follows.

CHAPTER 9

───── 🖎 ─────

Group Process: An Exploration of the True Self

Through years of working with cardiac patients from both the psychological and physiological perspective, I have repeatedly observed a pattern in many of my young, aggressive, Type-A, coronary-prone heart patients: they are preoccupied with performance issues, narcissistic drive and denial of feeling. Such maladaptive struggles create situations of isolation resulting in avoidance of intimacy. Many patients with heart disease have communicated to me deep feelings of loneliness. Fortunately, isolation and loneliness are two core issues that are highly responsive to group process.

In the beginning of this book, I discussed some of the principles of group therapy. Simply stated, in group situations one can connect to the feelings of another. Our attitudes, judgments and self-imposed belief systems frequently isolate us. Our thoughts can also close us off to others. In group process, however, it is more difficult to hide from our true feelings. A major goal of group experience is to help our patients discover the great wealth inherent in a healing community—empathy, compassion and forgiveness. The identification and expression of feelings are critical in breaking down the ego-driven Type-

209

A characteristics seen in these patients. Group process provides us the opportunity to see ourselves, our attitudes, beliefs and behaviors through others. In a safe and confidential psychotherapeutic environment, members are often surprised to find out what their true feelings really are. The most intense stressor that I know of is the disconnection of feeling (the heart) from thinking (the head). Such a disconnection can ultimately cause our demise as demonstrated by John Colter, the famous "mountain man" of the Lewis and Clark Expedition.

Colter was the best mountain man in the business. He was the best tracker, the best Indian fighter, the best there was in his profession. His life was the life of the wilderness.

One day in the early spring, he was out trapping on one of the tributaries of the Madison River with his associate, Mr. Potts. Suddenly, approximately 200 Indians surprised Colter. Potts raised a rifle, but before he could get the rifle up to his chest he was cut down by dozens of bullets and arrows. Potts was mortally wounded. Both men froze with fear as they were surrounded by Crow Indians. The Crow and Blackfeet tribes were enemies. Since Colter had previously fought on the side of the Blackfeet, he realized the danger of being face-to-face with the Crow.

Potts was captured and cut up into little pieces in front of Colter. Colter knew at this point that he was in serious trouble. He also knew that the Indians were playing a game with him. The chief then asked him how well he could run. Colter told the chief in Crow language that he was a "good runner." Colter was stripped naked. He was given a 200-yard head start. The chief took approximately 20 of his best braves with knives and hatchets. An arrow was shot in the air and the race was on.

Colter was running and running and running. Fortunately, he was in great shape. Without coverage for his feet, the prickly pear in the prairie pierced his soles. He was bleeding. He was spitting blood. He put forth an all-out effort, greater than 100 percent. He gave it everything he had. But, as he was running, he had this incredible insight. He knew that the Crow could not track well in water. A thought came into his mind. If he could make it to a tributary of the Madison River and get into the water, he might be able to escape. He was running hard. He was straining and gurgling when he made his agreement with God.

The agreement was very simple. He promised God that if he could get out of this one mess, just this one time, he would leave this God-forsaken territory, abandon trapping, quit being a mountain man, avoid any further expeditions and, perhaps, even get married and move to St. Louis. That was Colter's agreement with God.

John Colter was well into his sixth or seventh mile and literally so exhausted he was afraid to turn around. Suddenly he did turn and saw one brave behind him with a spear. Colter tripped. The young brave tried to kill him with his spear. Colter was somehow miraculously able to move away and subsequently killed his attacker. There were no other Indians in sight. Colter found the river and hid under a beaver embankment in the chilling water. Shortly after, he heard Indian braves all around him. After dark, he slipped out of the frozen water and escaped. He was found delirious 10 days later on the prairie, brought to an army fort and revived. He had survived!

Colter later wrote his memoirs including his recollection of his agreement with God. He moved to St. Louis, got married and had a baby. Now he suffered new stresses. He had to make a living, mend fences and pay taxes. Two years later Colter died suddenly of an infectious disease.

What killed John Colter? To the men who knew him, it was obvious. Colter's heart and passion was being a mountain man. As a result of his last close call, his head told him to move to civilization. Colter experienced the most severe stress there is. That is, his heart was saying one thing and his mind was saying another. His heart was drawn to the wilderness, his head rationalized civilization. He had become depressed and heartbroken. He had succumbed to an illness. In the end, his heart proved stronger than his will. Unfortunately, Colter did not follow the "voice" of his heart. He had lost his connection with his real passion.

Like John Colter, many of us often suffer a disconnection between our true feelings and our thoughts. Although individual psychotherapy can lead to personal growth, a group process experience with deep expression of feeling often supplies quicker resolution. Group process enhances awareness and consciousness. We are often able to receive the "truth" from others. In group therapy, exchange of energy among the participants helps to weave patterns of honesty.

An important concept of group process is not only how each member feels about himself, but also how members feel about one another. What we feel about others is often a reflection of our own issues in process, revealing more about us than about others. It is also important to note that the release of negativity and negative emotions can lead the group into an expression of tender feelings. It is an established fact, for example, that when the group leader does a "piece of work" on one person, perhaps focusing on shadow emotions of anger, negativity and rage, the cleansing reaction and emotional charge that occurs can literally open up the hearts of the entire group. This leads to the release of an enormous amount of energy, moving the group to a new level of awareness and insight. At these levels, new forms of healing take place arising from deep within our nature.

In healing the heart, we need to heal the core. In a safe environment where one is able to feel vulnerable in a space of total support, one has the potential to open up to his true feelings. Working with individuals on deep core issues frequently requires both cognitive and body-oriented therapy in order to go beyond the false self into true deep feelings. In order to break through denial and rigid patterns long entrenched in the personality, a total surrendering of the self is often a prerequisite. Individual psychotherapy, dyads (two people interacting) and group process can all be effective ways of discovering the true self while tapping into the unconscious attitudes of heartbreak. Uncovering issues of love and sexuality, which drive the essence of our characters, is also an essential ingredient in investigating our true nature.

Frequently, many questions are addressed in therapeutic group workshop situations. Some of these are:

1. What is the relationship between heartbreak and heart disease?
2. What is the connection between denial of feeling and cardiac disease?
3. Do power and control set the stage for the coronary-prone personality?
4. Do childhood longing and unmet needs create rules and attitudes that ultimately influence our adult lives?
5. Does the body remember what the mind forgets?
6. Do you dare to touch your own heartbreak?
7. Do you want to open your heart?
8. Do you want to touch your heart?

In our *Healing the Heart* training, different approaches and interventions are selected to help participants increase their own conscious awareness through making deeper contract with the unconscious aspects of themselves and others. Such trainings last four to six days, integrating psychological, emotional and spiritual healing. Various group process interventions, including bioenergetics, mental imagery, regression and meditation focus on the interaction between feelings, personality and character.

Healing the Heart Training

In an effort to understand the emotional and energetic factors of coronary-prone behavior, group therapy sessions are utilized to help individuals recognize established and frequently unsatisfactory behavioral responses to life situations. A primary goal in the "Healing the Heart Training" is the restoration of the person to a state of healthy pulsation or homeostasis. This work is accomplished experientially by exploring and balancing the energy of the autonomic nervous system.

As a result of cognitive and intensive body-oriented psychotherapy, participants deepen body awareness, particularly by exaggerating the already protracted sympathetic nervous system response. In the course of these workshops emphasis is placed on the recognition of self-destructive thinking patterns and on the expression and release of aggression and the "fight/flight" mechanism. The direction of such energy is channeled outward through such activities as acting out, aggression and the expression of negativity and struggle.

After participants struggle with issues of power and control through encounters with therapists, with one another in dyads and in groups, they are encouraged to explore the emotional counterpart of body contraction, energetic blocks and muscular contraction.

This state of sympathetic charge and discharge with subsequent physiological and emotional awareness is designed to give individuals considerable insight into their unconscious, autonomic sympathetic behavior patterns. During group process, many express being aware of profound feelings, blocked feelings or even no feeling. Even becoming aware of a lack of feeling or a block to feeling is an insight the individual needs to be able to move on to the next level—beginning to feel.

Utilizing special bioenergetic exercises such as grounding and falling, (see *Figure 4*, page 161) participants experience the sensation of letting down, letting go and giving in to struggle. Other processes focus on breathing, relaxation and meditation techniques. Participants begin to learn the process of "being" as opposed to "doing" as they learn to surrender and trust. Falling exercises are utilized in group situations, creating a bridge between the two opposing arms of the nervous system, one of being vigilant and holding oneself up and the other of surrender into feeling or being.

Falling bioenergetic maneuvers place stress on the lower extremities, which eventually results in a softening and letting down of the body armoring. By placing all the weight on one leg, slightly bent at the knee, the individual eventually falls. How long the person maintains this painful stance in spite of the invitation to "let go" when ready is an additional insight into the level or degree of ego investment and determination involved in never allowing the self to "give up" or let down. Some of my competitive, driven, coronary patients have withstood amazingly long periods of pain to "hold their ground" and resist surrender. This particular exercise has provided them an incredible awareness of the extent to which they will disconnect from their true self or feeling (pain) to maintain the false self's performance that "I can take it!" It is eventually a relief to them to begin to let go of the defensive ego investment that has consumed so much of their energy in their adult life and begin to surrender into their own softness.

The contact and withdrawal involved in such a maneuver allows the participants to experience a sense of failure eliciting feelings of worthlessness and loss of self-esteem. These emotions, frequently denied by coronary-prone individuals, are accepted without judgment in a group setting of tremendous emotional support. In order to experience joy, one must be able to be free of anxieties about failing, softening, feeling and expressing emotion.

How Have I Hurt You?

In addition to group process maneuvers, experiential dyads are also quite helpful in the mobilization of emotion, aggression, contact and awareness. The "How Have I Hurt You" dyad is useful in the investigation of our unconscious feelings of heartbreak, the cardinal emotion frequently denied by the person with coronary heart disease. In this process two people, A and B, face each other. There is no talking during this process unless so instructed by the group leader. After making eye contract with one another, A offers B the words, "How have I hurt you?"

Continued eye contact is made and the words, "How have I hurt you" are delivered over and over again. Whatever feelings come up are all encouraged. After a few more minutes of eye contact and expression of feeling, A turns to B offering the words, "I am so sorry for wounding you." B is now given the opportunity to take this gesture in and feel whatever emotion is associated with that statement. Continued eye contact is made while the phrase is delivered several times. After the process is over, A and B share their experience with one another. After a few minutes of sharing, the experience can be repeated with a reversal of roles. Changing partners is also permissible. This simple process often begins to break down the enormous denial around one's heartbreak. Anger, sadness, shame and rage have been elicited by such interactions. The dyad is not only useful for the awareness it brings but also in the way it allows access to the polarity of the "dark side."

Following this exercise, a heart meditation using imagery, touch and a metaphorical inner healer allows each participant to make deeper contact with himself and others. The meditation is then followed by another dyad focusing on simple contact, vulnerability and intimacy.

The space created by this exercise allows for the possibility of softer feelings of vulnerability to emerge in a contact and withdrawal dyad. One's negativity is released without retaliation or judgment. The experience of a space conducive for soft simple contact follows the expression of negativity.

Simple Contact

Again, this is a nonverbal dyad interaction. Eye contact, arm contact, shoulder contact and eventually, head to head contact with awareness of breathing now ground the individuals into a safe space where soft, nonsexual contact and withdrawal of contact are experienced. The awareness in this exercise focuses the immediate feelings associated with soft, simple contact and the withdrawal of that touch. These two dyads and group process meditation are ways of exploring the connection between unconscious vs. conscious drives.

Yoga, meditation and guided imagery are other useful interventions that may reduce sympathetic tone while facilitating the journey out of the head and into the body. The regression process, a profound meditative and body-oriented experience, unveils early childhood experiences in order to take the individual to an even deeper level of self awareness.

Regression Encounter Process

This maneuver lasts approximately two hours and may help the patient reexperience the pain of childhood heartbreak. Developmentally, as noted, this heartbreak occurs less frequently during infancy and more often between the ages of four and six, the Oedipal period of one's life. Just prior to this exercise, the participants are engaged in charging the sympathetic nervous system. This is done through experiencing negativity, utilizing temper tantrums, verbal and physical protest, kicking and performing actions to release pent-up anger and rage and charge up the sympathetic nervous system. Following the process, the participants are asked to lie down on the floor and connect to the feelings evoked in their body.

Next, after a meditative process focusing on complete body relaxation, participants are asked to imagine themselves as the director of a play called *This is Your Life*. They are taken back from the present situation in stages of five- to ten-year increments to when they were six months of age. The process is very detailed as they go back through the regression. They are questioned about what decisions they have made in their lives and what they are experiencing in their bodies as they go back in time. The regression process is very powerful. Following the process, participants may experience a complete discharge of energy.

The energy in the room can be quite moving, very charged with positive feelings. People feel young, vulnerable and close to one another. They often hold out their hands, reaching out and allowing themselves to be touched or held. They reexperience their earlier and current heartbreak with support and often report this to be a powerful cleansing experience.

Such heartbreak feelings originating in infancy, Oedipal periods and adolescence gradually emerge allowing participants to become aware, perhaps for the very first time, that early childhood defenses (deadening of feeling, use of power to overcome pain and humiliation, closed heart feelings and suppressed emotions) have become adult maladaptive personality characteristics with the potential to affect their heart and health. In general, none of us really want to experience the psychic pain of heartbreak, helplessness and humiliation that we encountered in childhood. To reexamine such feelings places us in seemingly life-threatening situations, since as children we all had the feeling that we could actually die if we truly took in all of what we were feeling. Thus, for many of us, denial of this "death-layer" experience is preferable to reconnecting with the self. In our workshops, however, participants are hungry for insight into their present situations.

The energy is so positive, so high that they become willing to risk taking on this challenging experience.

This profound process yields tremendous awareness for many attending the "Healing the Heart" workshops. A good physician or therapist must be able to redirect the internal energies of the patient toward his or her own healing. Although the healer needs to nourish that power within, it is the patient's openness to therapy that is the most important aspect in healing. Group process is one way to open the door to the unconscious.

*   *   *

Over the decades, Freud suggested that remembering childhood experiences had no curative effect unless suppressed emotions are revealed. He suggested the word "resistance," which was the patient's inability to experience early suppressed emotions. A few years later in *Character Analysis*, Reich discussed the elaborate defense systems that patients construct to protect themselves from the outside world as well as from their own feelings. He viewed the human being as a unified system rather than a distinct composite of psyche and soma. He theorized that when a person denies his or her emotions, the disruption of the flow of energy converts into physical and emotional blocks. These blocks are manifested in the armoring of the body and reveal themselves in how the individuals hold and move the body. These blocks also set the stage for stagnation of the normal healthy pulsation and flow of energy.

Lowen's theory, which incorporates emotional conflict with physical body expression, appealed to me as a cardiologist. Because breathing is the major factor supplying energy to the body, Lowen maintains that breathing should be used, not only as a technique to release feeling, but also as a means of developing deeper, fuller, life-giving respirations. I agree wholeheartedly with this concept. Deeper breathing is not only essential in healing the heart, but is also a major goal in the therapeutic process of enhancing pulsation.

"Healing the Heart" is about the restoration of energy within the heart and, therefore, the self. It is about redirecting and preserving the energy of the body, mind and spirit. To begin such a journey, one needs to understand the truth of the body. An Eastern philosopher put it this way: "The man who realizes the truth of the body can then come to know the truth of the universe." The pulsatory movement of our life force is directly connected to the pulsatile vibratory energy of the universe; to know the body is to know the difference between the suppressed pain of chronic contraction and the joy of full expansion and expression.

The goal of psychotherapy, group process and bioenergetic integration involves insight, self-awareness, the release of tension and the connection of body to mind. When such an integration occurs, the body becomes graceful. Graceful movements are not ego-directed, nor are they willed. Graceful movements are usually not in the domain of the excessive drive and struggle encountered in the coronary-prone narcissistic character.

The coronary-prone personality projects to the outside world the false image of power and strength. Depression or a sense of inner emptiness is the price he or she pays for the energy-exhausting maintenance of this image. Living in such a false self does not allow for an investment in true deep feeling. The false self cannot experience fullness in life because it is really a cover-up for the secrets we hide. Narcissism is an unconscious defensive strategy for maintaining this cover-up. Narcissistic behavior is governed by attitudes, rules, judgment and self-aggrandizement. As the narcissistic character unveils the false image and begins to experience the real self, he or she begins the path to the truth which can lead to spiritual awakening and joy. Opening one's heart and getting in touch with true deep feeling allows one to experience who he or she really is. When the false self is shed, one gives up his or her image and, in turn, the life-long struggle of loneliness and isolation.

Group process analysis opens the way to this understanding. This awareness and insight begins the process of self-discovery which builds the platform for a new spiritual opportunity. This is the true essence of healing. All the answers are within ourselves. We are now ready to explore the next and highest level of healing—the spiritual nature of heart disease.

Chapter 10

——— ✍ ———

Spirituality and the Heart

So far, we have considered many approaches to healing the heart. Unquestionably, they are all important. Diet, nutritional supplementation, exercise, proper breathing and healthy release of emotional, physical and sexual energy all play an integral part in reestablishing and maintaining the vitality of the heart. In addition, the nurturing of loving and supportive relationships has a tremendous positive impact on the quality of our lives. Psychotherapy and body-oriented therapies may also take us to even deeper levels of awareness and insight. But there is another element to the healing process which binds these multiple threads together and weaves them back into the seamless fabric of human life. That element is the life of the spirit. There are an increasing number of cardiologists, psychotherapists and other mind/body therapists who are counseling heart patients about the amazing untapped potential of spiritual power that can be employed in the prevention and treatment of heart disease. More and more "prescriptions" include group process, prayer, the practice of forgiveness, trust in a divine power and the pursuit of a spiritual connection. A sense of community connection with spirituality may also be gained by attending a church or synagogue.

What is spirituality? Is it organized religion, that is, going

222

to church every Sunday or to Temple on specific holidays? Is it sitting in a lotus position, completely absorbed in some transcendental meditation? Is it searching for a guru? Or is it belonging to a group or cult that shares a similar belief system? While spirituality may embrace any of these, each of us must follow our own unique pathway to spirituality.

Spirituality is a journey that each of us has the capacity to embark upon. It is a crucial component of each person's life. Throughout this book, I have been discussing mind, body and spirit connections. We can see and touch the body and think about both body and mind in physiological and psychological terms. The spirit, however, is less knowable even though it is the link that joins body and mind to function as a whole. Without spirit, there can be no growth or direction.

Spirituality doesn't mean you have to believe in the conventional notion of God or to go to religious services regularly. I believe spirituality is each person's set of beliefs about a power outside of himself. It is having faith in that power and turning to it for courage, strength and direction. You may be asking yourself, aren't religion and spirituality the same thing? The very word religion means to relink, to bind, to reconnect. However, the concept of spirituality is more metaphorical than that of religion. It is the theoretical framework upon which religions base their facts, dogma and faith. Religions are organized to explain, harness and elaborate on the underlying spiritual premise. Although religion is one pathway to the spiritual domain, the essence of spirituality goes beyond religion. It is the individual who makes the final leap of faith. When this happens, spirituality can relink or reconnect body and mind, matter and spirit and man and God.

You may be wondering why a cardiologist is advocating spirituality. Aren't medicine and spirituality opposite sides of the spectrum? One is grounded in concrete knowledge of the physical, the other in faith. Actually, I believe that medical treatment is as much about your belief that you can really heal yourself as it is about surgeries and drugs.

For example, in medicine we sometimes use the term "placebo effect" to describe an outcome which is attributed to one's expectations or beliefs about a drug effect as opposed to the actual action of the drug. If a person has a belief in the power of a drug or an overwhelming optimism that the drug will work, positive expectancy is created. With this positive expectancy, we know that the drug is more likely to work. This leads us to ponder, what are the forces that heal? Is it pharmacotherapy or is it placebo effect? Or, is it both? It is an established fact that our emotions have the potential to create the physiology of healing. Spirituality can also heal us. For many, positive links do exist between spiritual practice and healing the heart. We will now consider some of the methods of bolstering heart health with spirit.

Appreciation of connection and surrender to something greater than one's self is really the essence of spirituality. For example, in a previous chapter, we looked into the power of meditation. Meditation can lead you out of your head and into your body. When we establish a deep and relaxed breathing style, our body becomes relaxed. When thoughts arise, we just notice them but don't get caught up in them. When we are in this state, we can then use visualization to ask for guidance from a spiritual power in which we believe. We may ask a spiritual figure for an answer. When a message comes, we trust that metaphorically, it is taking root inside of our heart. The heart is, indeed, the core of the body. It is also the spiritual center. We have all heard how a spiritual insight or connection can literally "lift our heart" by giving us an experience of transcendence. In this regard, meditation is very close to prayer. Like meditation, prayer can alter our body and transcend us into another dimension. We must never underestimate the power of prayer not only as a healing modality, but also as another way of making a connection with something greater than the self.

Prayer

The difference between prayer and meditation is subtle. In meditation, we quiet ourselves to access our inner healer or voice and "listen" for an answer. Some of us may even ask God to come to us in meditation. When we pray, we reach beyond ourselves to offer our prayers up to God. It is important to remember to pray for the health of our hearts as well as our souls.

Because heart disease is often a life-threatening problem, it is not surprising that many heart patients turn to their faith and pray to a higher power for healing. In a previous chapter, I discussed the case of Mary for whom thousands of people across the state of Connecticut were praying. She survived. Did community prayer affect Mary's outcome? I believe it did.

From the beginning of time, our ancestors often assumed that faith and healing were interrelated. It has only been in the last couple of centuries, with the intervention of the scientific method, that we decided that things which could not be scientifically proven were somehow "not real." Actually, the separation of science and spirituality occurred in the 17th century when philosopher René Descartes struck a deal with the Catholic Church. Matters concerning the body and the physical world were put into the hands of science to dissect, explore and explain. But matters of religion, the spirit, the mind, the emotions and mortality remained in the domain of the church.

We now know that is futile to try to separate the mind from the body, the spirit from the mind, or the heart from any other part of the human organism. The scientific method is nothing more than a process of watching what happens in a controlled situation, then drawing conclusions about the results. Over the centuries, such divisive patterns have undermined the connection between body and soul. Recently, medical science has begun to apply the scientific method to a study of prayer.

In *Healing Words,* Larry Dossey describes prayer as an act in which an individual makes contact with a higher power. Dr. Dossey describes many studies that demonstrate how prayer has evoked physical healing, not only among people praying for themselves, but among people who have been prayed for by others. Dossey describes the work of cardiologist Randolph Byrd who studied a group of 393 patients at San Francisco General Hospital. In this study, participants were randomly assigned to two groups by computer. Half were prayed for and half were not. The patients in the prayed-for group were "five times less likely to require antibiotics, three times less likely to develop severe heart failure." None of the prayed-for group required the assistance of a respirator compared to 12 in the control group.

In a smaller study at a London Clinic, 38 rheumatoid arthritic patients were divided into two groups. Half were prayed for, although they didn't know it, and half were not. Of the six patients who improved, five were in the prayed-for group. In another small study involving 18 children with leukemia, 10 were prayed for by anonymous individuals and 8 were not. Of the 10 in the prayed-for group, 7 were still alive after 15 months, compared to just 2 out of 8 children in the other group. Prayer is indeed a powerful medium in healing.

Dossey believes that petitionary prayer, in which people seek support from their personal God or higher power, nourishes a spiritual connection. It is when we surrender to something higher and greater than ourselves that our life assumes a greater purpose. When life is enriched by a sense of profound purpose, our perspective is shifted, offering a deeper meaning in the challenges that confront us in our daily lives including heart disease. As a cardiologist, I frequently encourage my patients to pray. Even in the most serious of circumstances, I often offer my patients renewed hope and strength through prayer. In times of crisis, I have also been blessed to experience deep connections with my patients while praying together. Praying is an enriching experience that can extend us beyond ourselves. Moreover, prayer requires contemplation.

Contemplation offers time to ponder the nature of the divine as well as our place as individuals in the complexity of a larger life scheme. Contemplation is another way of surrendering to something greater than ourselves. One of the ways we can retreat from the world is returning to nature. Let me tell you about a recent Alaskan fishing trip which I took with my family.

Nature

During the first three weeks in August of 1995, I participated in a fishing adventure with my brother and my two sons. Although the fishing was absolutely wonderful, the Alaskan adventure meant much more to me. First of all, I found myself thanking God for giving me the opportunity to spend such precious time with my family. I also found that hiking in the forest, fishing in the streams, watching the eagles in the trees and sharing the habitat with bears and wolves helped me to reconnect with my own body and its feelings. After hours of fishing to the rhythmic motion of casting, I occasionally found myself praying to a higher power. I wasn't focused on doing; I was just being.

Why is this connectedness with your loved ones and your body an embodiment of spirit? Many of us feel happiness in the presence of people with whom we really wish to be. Interacting with loved ones creates a positive energy that springs from feelings of love. This connectedness enhances our well-being and joy. These feelings cannot be explained intellectually. They originate deep inside of us and are a tremendous source of nurturance, peace and tranquility. These are, in fact, spiritual feelings. On this wilderness trip I found that being close to my family while pursuing my own activities sparked spiritual feelings in me.

Look at your own life and think about which things make you feel connected to others and to the rest of the world; which experiences make you feel spiritual? Write them down and plan to do them more often. They will help put you onto a spiritual path to healing your heart.

Journaling and Reading

Writing a journal is one of the best ways to deepen your connection with yourself and keep yourself on a spiritual path. I know people who keep a prayer journal. They pray regularly, write down what they pray for and how their prayers are answered. Some of you may resist attempting an exercise like this. Let me offer you a suggestion. If you can't think about anything else to write, write about your writing block. You will find that writing quickly disassociates your internal critic from your true inner voice, allowing you full expression of that which you have been holding back. When you have completed this nonjudgmental writing, spend a few minutes reflecting on what you have learned. I know that when I write books, newsletters or journal articles, much of what I write about is an extension of my unconscious self. You can use your own journal to record discoveries, breakthroughs and milestones along your road to spirituality and health. Writing a journal is a great form of contemplation because you are spending time with yourself.

Reading spiritual and inspirational materials will also help you to contemplate and reflect on your true self. There is a tremendous array of inspiring books in bookstores these days, which probably reflects our general need to reconnect with our spirituality. There are wonderful books with daily meditations and reflections including the Holy Bible, the Torah and the Koran. Browse through any of these books and you will find something that appeals to you. In addition, there are many works available by saints and mystics. It is valuable to expose yourself to a variety of viewpoints because each one offers a unique insight and its own particular message.

For example, I remember one important message I received from one of my patients who was dying from cancer. It was during the Christmas holidays. His words were, "In the light of eternity, what does it matter?" From a dying patient, these words were true to my own heart. It is a message that I will never forget and I often call it to my mind during crisis periods in my own life. Meditation, prayer and contemplation are all ways to experience spirituality. Another vehicle to facilitate the presence and connection of spirit is music.

Music

Let music into your life. Music can access our spiritual center in a way that nothing else can. The next time you are caught in a rush hour traffic, turn off the radio and plug in a tape or CD of Pachelbel's Canon or a Gregorian Chant. It is important to note how the music of meditation can slow us down and bring us back to our center. Relaxing to music not only deepens our breathing, but also opens our heart. Music also gives us permission to surrender.

The ability to surrender is perhaps the most difficult step for any cardiac patient to take. A heart attack is one way which literally forces a patient to surrender. When we surrender, we place ourselves in the hands of others. But the ultimate surrender is "not my will, but thine." Through the act of surrendering, we open ourselves to more spiritual forces; we realize that something greater than ourselves is in charge here. The trick to surrendering is to get the ego (which likes to think it is in charge) out of the way, so the spirit can work its way through into our human life. One way of surrendering is to forgive.

Forgiveness

Anger, hostility and resentment block us from spirituality. Forgiveness is a way to transcend hostility. Hostility is often manifested as a cynical view of the world. When you are free of toxic hostility you are more connected to others. By learning to forgive, we can move to a different level, approaching a more spiritual attitude. Simply stated, forgiveness means letting go of the past. The negative energy we hold from past events insidiously attacks our spirituality and our physical bodies as well.

Let me give you an example. Earlier I discussed the feelings that arose when I was sued for medical malpractice many years ago. During the lawsuit, my back suddenly went out. The trial was literally "breaking my back." I developed two bulging discs and for several years thereafter I continued to have lower back pain. Eventually, my back discomfort became so severe that I had difficulty walking, sitting and carrying out daily activities. I sought many healing modalities. I saw physical therapists, psychotherapists, acupuncturists, orthopedic surgeons and continued my program in intense rolfing. However, it was not until I sought the services of a spiritual therapist that my path to healing really began. It was truly fortuitous.

I had been working on a chapter of my second book with Ellen, a metaphysical spiritual psychotherapist. I told her about my back discomfort and its historical and emotional roots. She intuitively counseled me that in order to heal my back, I needed to grant forgiveness to the people who had falsely accused me. Following a deep meditation, she helped me to visualize the family who had "injured" me. She then asked that I honestly acknowledge to myself how much I had been hurt. She was clear that I was not to overdramatize the situation or place blame on anyone. Following this exercise, she asked that I see if I could find a place in my heart to forgive unconditionally. As she worked with me to forgive the family who had sued me, she gently and supportively placed her hand on my back, focusing my energy to bring the forgiveness down to the lower spine.

Although I only participated in one forgiveness meditative exercise with Ellen, the discomfort in my back improved at least 50 percent. I was able to walk without the previous twist in my alignment. A resentful back, like a resentful heart, creates a trapped negative energy field that is on its way to some form of dis-ease. Sometimes you need to forgive before you can heal. If it is impossible for you to receive or seek forgiveness for something that has been troubling you, consider working with a therapist or spiritual counselor.

Resentments or deep hostilities can literally keep us on the hook. When we can gently release resentments, we have made a large stride in healing. Granting forgiveness to someone who has injured you is as important as seeking forgiveness from another that you may have injured. There is a big difference between apologizing and asking for forgiveness. Simply saying "I'm sorry" doesn't go far enough for serious offenses; it can be self-righteous, arrogant and presumptive, not to mention ineffective. Some of us have deeply wounded others. In the process of asking for forgiveness, we may need to ask God to give us courage.

Seeking forgiveness from another is surrendering the part of you which participated in the creation of a wound. Before we can solicit forgiveness from another, we have to acknowledge and honor that feeling in the injured party. After recognizing the feelings that are present, we must allow the injured party to express his or her anger, hurt and negativity. It is very important that we try not to rationalize or defend our participation in the past wounding of another. After encouraging the expression of negativity, we need to take responsibility for our own part. After acknowledging the responsibility we have had in causing this wound, a heartfelt apology must follow. When we are able to apologize with humility and sincerity, we come from a place of vulnerability. Although we need to accept the possibility of rejection, the fact remains that after a meaningful dialogue with the injured party a heart-felt "I'm sorry" may be the most healing words we can say. When we can say the words "I am so sorry," the heart opens up not only to an emotional place but also a spiritual place. Opening the heart to yourself and others is a way to strengthen your heart.

Let me tell you about two opening-the-heart stories in my practice of cardiology and psychotherapy.

Ron Smith

Ron was undergoing emergency bypass surgery. His family waited patiently and in great fear about his survival. Eventually, the surgeon emerged from the operating room with a smile on his face. He took the hands of Ron's wife into his own to reassure her that things had gone well. "Your husband is going to make it. He'll be okay." Ron's daughter, an artist, turned to her mother as the surgeon walked away. "Mom, you just held the hands of the man who touched Dad's heart." Even as I write this now, I feel the tears well up in my eyes. Sometimes it takes surgery to literally open your heart to yourself and others.

Ron was a typical "Type-A" personality, totally absorbed in his work. There was little room for other people in his life since his job consumed all his energies. As an engineer, and an excellent one at that, he was working on a large project for a major aircraft manufacturing company, sometimes working seven days a week. The job was extremely stressful. Management was under pressure to cut costs and Ron felt that many demands were expected of him without the resources to back him up.

One Saturday afternoon, as he was mowing his lawn, Ron became short of breath. After seeing his family doctor, he was instructed to see a cardiologist right away. I still remember the day that Ron walked into my office. Ron's history was classic and his symptoms had increased steadily. I looked him in the eye and told him, "You have major blockages in your arteries. You need to be hospitalized right now."

Ron trustingly took my advice, knowing that my expertise was hearts just as his was jet engines. During an arteriogram, a procedure which lights up the coronary vessels, Ron's anatomy showed life-threatening blockages requiring emergency surgery. Ron recovered fully and a week following surgery returned to my office. Now, the *real* healing began.

I told Ron that he had "bypassed' his heart problem. We then talked about what his life was like before surgery. I knew Ron was an intelligent man. He had a great deal of insight and I asked him if he thought his heart disease was inevitable. I asked him if heart disease could be a "gift in disguise" or if the experience of his emergency surgery could be a messenger of something more? Ron listened attentively. He suddenly "got it." I felt a deep connection between the two of us. And I felt in my heart that Ron was ready to change his life.

I treated Ron on two levels, one physical and the other psychological. Ron realized the true "message" in his heart disease, and he participated in our cardiac rehabilitation groups and couples group. He talked about his experience with others. He told people how the attachment to his job had run his life. As a workaholic, there had been no room for anything else. His heart had not been open to family, friends or even to his own feelings. We explored further the reasons Ron had heart disease since he was not the typical profile. Ron was tall, slim, did not smoke or drink and ate a very healthy diet. Ron's major risk factor was the denial of the stress in his life. He responded to work pressures by running faster and working harder. He was preoccupied by performing, meeting deadlines and meeting the needs of both upper and lower management. He had been desperately trapped, but he hadn't known it.

Maladaptive struggles create situations of isolation, resulting in avoidance of intimacy and contact with friends, family and even a higher power. At the time of Ron's illness he was the deacon of his church. Although he had a strong spiritual connection, prayed and read the Bible, Ron's attachment to his job determined his priorities. That is, family and God had become displaced by the incessant demands of the job. The pressures of work took Ron away from the things that were truly precious to his heart. I believe that evil or Satanic forces can get hooks into us through our workaholic tendencies. In this day and age it is easy to be seduced into over-performance by financial insecurity, uncertainty of the times and even our own ego needs. Although Ron attempted to relieve some of his job stress by trying to talk to his superiors, they refused to listen. Ron saw no escape from his situation. His only way out was to die or develop an illness. Fortunately he chose the latter.

Following his surgery and weeks of rehabilitation, Ron went back to work with a new enthusiasm and outlook on life. But after approximately 10 months of being in the pressure cooker Ron had the intuitive feeling that he could get sick again. This time he made the conscious decision that he was not going to die for his job. He looked deeper into his emotional and spiritual self. An early retirement package was being offered and Ron decided to take it. He sold his house and moved to a small Vermont college town to be closer to his sons.

It was "heart" and heart disease that really changed Ron's life, because he listened to the spiritual message. Following his bypass surgery, he had a spiritual rebirth. A surgeon had opened his chest, but it was Ron who had opened his heart.

With his wife, sons, daughter and friends rallying around him, he emerged from his personal crisis realizing how many people loved him. With so much positive support, Ron experienced a spiritual awakening, made a choice and transformed his whole life. With such a massive reframing he was able to see everything in his life more clearly. He listened to the message of his heart disease and took responsibility to turn his life around. Today Ron feels his life is fuller than it ever was—closer to nature, and closer in his relationships with his wife, his children and with God.

What can we learn from Ron's story? Is there a message for all of us? Ron's story indeed has a happy ending. And remember it was Ron's choices that affected his health. It was his choice of lifestyle, belief systems, relationships and belief in a higher spiritual power that brought Ron into true physical healing—the integration of his body, mind and spirit. Ron also had the belief that he could get well and he did get well. He knew that the stress of his job could kill him. Ron accepted things as they were and made the choice to get better. I'm not recommending that everyone quit his job, move to the country and become spiritual. What I am saying is that if we heed our own personal messengers and make choices based on our intuition and spiritual perceptions, our lives will unfold in a positive way.

Research suggests that people who do get well despite life-threatening illnesses such as cancer and heart disease are more assertive, even aggressive with physicians, healthcare workers and employers to negotiate treatments, recovery and even their future. In order to get well, we must fight back.

Although it is extremely important to be in control and make choices, overcontrol can be the Achilles heel for every one of us. We must listen to the messages around us and surrender. It may seem paradoxical, but to be truly in control, we must be willing to let go. The one who trusts, believes in himself or herself and has faith can surrender more easily.

When a devastating illness slaps us in the face, we have to make choices. It is our responsibility to act on those choices, even if it requires some risk. Maybe this is one of the hidden benefits of heart disease. Perhaps, if you really listen to what's going on around you the way Ron Smith did, heart disease can help change the way you live your life. For many of my patients, heart disease *has* given them an opportunity to look at the way they choose to live in the world. After taking an honest look at his life, Ron committed to what really had true meaning for him. He decided to stop and smell the roses.

Bob Hay, another of my exceptional heart patients, used his heart disease as a way to complete all the relationships he had in his life.

"He brought it upon himself." If ever that saying about self-destructive behavior applied to anyone, it was my patient Bob Hay.

Bob Hay

Bob suffered a heart attack and had coronary bypass surgery, yet he continued to smoke and to work at his stressful job. By the time he retired, quit cigarettes and cut down on his fat intake, the fluid had built up in his chest to the point that he could not even bend over to tie his own shoes. He couldn't even walk across the room; his quality of life was terrible. He was so full of anger and rage.

I told Bob that if he could direct his rage into healing himself, he had a chance to live. Otherwise, he would soon need a heart transplant. Bob and his wife Frances began to attend my heart health workshops. He slowly opened up to others and began to confront the anger that had been driving many of his self-destructive actions. He learned to breathe properly, to relax and meditate and to share his feelings with other group members. The real turning point for Bob came when he realized if he did not drastically improve his health, a day would come when Frances would wake up or come home from work and find him dead. He had resigned himself to the damage done to his own body by his self-destructive behavior, but the idea of causing grief and pain to Frances was more than he could bear. He finally resolved to get better.

With the help of his wife, Bob had not smoked a cigarette in three years. He has lost 25 pounds on a healthy diet including fruits, vegetables, grains, fish and chicken. He took coenzyme Q_{10} and other nutritional supplements. Although he had numerous episodes of congestive heart failure and required oxygen to breathe, his heart's pumping efficiency improved. In my heart health workshops, Bob started setting goals to give himself a reason to keep on living. At first, he wanted to see his daughter graduate from college. He attended the graduation. In another workshop, Bob told the group that his youngest daughter had a baby with a man she hadn't married. This was offensive to Bob's moral values. Because of the rigidity of his thinking, there was an irreparable rift in their relationship.

In the Healing the Heart workshops, we worked on Bob's rage and anger. Underneath these feelings was a deeper layer of sadness and sorrow. As Bob shared his sorrows with other group members, he began to cry deeply. Such crying was healing to his own heart as well as healing to the relationship with his daughter. He told the group that when he first saw his grandchild, he just fell apart. He threw out his previous moral standards, reembraced his daughter and began to nurture the relationship. He felt that he had a new outlook on life. He was more respectful of people and found a new empathy in ways he had never experienced.

Unfortunately, in the summer of 1995, after several surgeries due to the complications of diabetes, Bob died at home. Although he knew he might die from the damage he had inflicted on his body, the changes he was able to make in the last years of his life gave those years a richness and poignancy that otherwise might never have happened.

In other words, it was Bob's struggle with heart disease which really made him look at his life. His relationships deepened. He became an inspiration to those around him. His courage to tell the truth in our group workshops was an inspiration to many others. Although he has passed on, he continues to live in the hearts and the memories of his family and friends. He lives in my heart and mind as one of the most exceptional patients I have ever known. He lives in those who hear his story and use it as a motivation to change their own lives. And I would like to believe that he lives on in the ebb and flow of the spiritual life that contains and sustains us all.

The path of healing the heart will not give us immortality, only the life of the spirit can give us that. But if we take the first step, the divine will move closer to us in response. Another of my patients, George Kingsbury, expressed this in one of my workshops. After a meditation, I asked the participants to seek guidance from a wise healer or a religious figure. During the process, a message came to George. In an interview with writer Henry Dreher, George said the following:

> I was a strong believer that there is a God and an order of things. But, between Steve's workshop and the reading I have done, I see where I have made some mistakes as far as my personal beliefs are concerned. I always thought that if you work hard and try to do the right thing, everything would be okay. Now I understand that God isn't going to come to me, no matter how good I am. I am going to have to go to Him."

Going to God, for George, made all of the difference, not just in his mental outlook, but also in his physical health and well-being. For George, the step toward spirituality sparked his physical healing.

Health is not just a condition of the physical body but also a condition of mind, divine spirit, love and truth. When we accept this, our body rests in a state of balance where real healing is possible. When we embrace the healing trinity of body, mind and spirit, we can truly embrace pulsation and eventually grace. This is the basis and essence of optimum health and freedom from disease.

My patients have taught me so much about the preciousness of life. If you want to heal or prevent heart disease, the first step is recognition of old wounds, losses and your emotional reactions to them. The next step is mobilizing those trapped energies and feelings and discharging them in ways that are nurturing to your heart. Following a healthy lifestyle is another significant step toward obtaining optimum health. The final step in healing is to realize the profound depth of spirituality and how heart disease can, indeed, be a messenger of something more.

On some level we have all experienced heartbreak in our lives. We know that in susceptible individuals heartbreak can set the stage for heart disease. Although we may not own it, every one of us possesses a deep dark side. We also know that our patterns of thought, behavior and our styles of communication determine the quality of our relationships. They can be fulfilling or they can be marred by frustration and alienation.

Alienation is the root of that unholy trinity of coronary-prone Type-A characteristics—hostility, cynicism and self-absorption. Our unconscious mind-set also determines our internal biochemical and physiological reactions. Subtle, long-term internal changes undermine health and well-being and when combined with patterns of maladaptive behavior create a self-perpetuating, downward spiraling cascade of events which can ultimately prove fatal. Heart disease has offered many of my patients an opportunity to reflect on their lives.

I do not believe the heart is just a mechanical pump that moves blood through our bodies. It holds a deeper meaning as the metaphorical center of our spiritual life. To me, the heart is a flaming crimson jewel, a pulsating universal star that beats to the rhythm of our lives. It can pulse in time to the chaos of the world around us or it can beat in time with the pulsations of the divine. The voice of the heart can often lead us to the truth, not always an easy journey. Sometimes an illness like heart disease is placed in our path for a specific reason. In the final analysis, we need to look for the message our wounded heart is bringing us; we need to ponder deeply the true essence of our lives.

Bibliography

Chapter 1

Epstein , G. *Healing Immortality.* New York: Bantam, 1994.

Epstein, G. *Healing Visualization.* New York: Bantam, 1989.

Eisenberg, D. M, et al. Unconventional Medicine in the United States: Prevalence, Costs, and Patterns of Use 1993;328:246-252.

Eliot, R. S., and D. L. Breo. *Is It Worth Dying For?* New York: Bantam, 1984.

Lowen, A. *Love, Sex and Your Heart.* New York: Macmillan, 1988.

Miller, A. *Prisoners of Childhood* New York: Basic Books, 1981.

Peabody, F. The Care of the Patient. *JAMA* 1927; 88: 877–82

Peck, M. S. *The Road Less Traveled* New York: Simon & Schuster, 1978.

Peck, M. S. *People of the Lie.* New York: Simon & Schuster, 1983.

Pelletier, K. *Sound Mind, Sound Body..* New York: Simon & Schuster, 1994.

Pelletier, K. *Mind as Healer, Mind as Slayer.* New York: Dell, 1977.

Siegel, B. S. *Peace, Love and Healing.* New York: Harper & Row, 1989.

Sinatra, S. T. *Optimum Health* New York: Lincoln Bradley, 1996.

Chapter 2

Friedman, M, and Rosenman, R. *Type A Behavior and Your Heart.* New York: Fawcett, 1974.

Lynch, J. *The Language of the Heart: The Human Body in Dialogue.* New York: Basic Books, 1985.

Lynch, J. *The Broken Heart.* New York: Basic Books, 1977.

Reich, W. *Character Analysis.* New York: Farrar, Straus & Giroux, 1945.

Ruberman, W, E. et al. Psychosocial Influences on Mortality after Myocardial Infarction. *N Engl J Med* 1984;311:552-559.

Santoriski, J. Letting the Heart Breathe. In D. Boadella, ed., *Energy and Character.* London: Abbotsbury Publications, B.C.M. 1985 (1-23).

Sinatra, S. T, and A. Lowen. Heartbreak and Heart Disease—The Origin and Essence of Coronary-Prone Behavior. *Holistic Medicine* 1987;2:169-172.

Sinatra, S. T. Stress and the Heart—Behavioral Interactions and Plan for Strategy. *Conn Medicine* 1984; 48:81-86.

Chapter 3

Cannon, W. B. Voodoo Death. *Psychosomatic Medicine* 1957;19:182-190.
Cannon, W. B. Stresses and Strains of Homeostasis. *Am J Med Science* 1935;189:1-14.
Deanfield J. E. et al. Clinical Evaluation of Transient Myocardial Ischemia During Daily Life. *Am J Med* 1985;79:18-24.
Lowen, A. *Narcissism: The Denial of Feeling.* New York: Macmillan Publishing, 1985.
Lowen, A. *Pleasure,* New York: Penguin, 1975.
Selye, H. *Stress in Health and Disease.* Boston: Butterworth, Inc., 1976.
Selye, H. *The Physiology and Pathology of Exposure to Stress.* Montreal: Acta, Inc. 1950.
Sinatra, S. T. and L. A. Feitell. The Heart and Mental Stress, Real and Imagined. *Lancet* 222-223, 1985.
Sinatra, S. T. et al. A Stress Management Seminar with Biochemical Assay. *Conn Medicine* 1982;46(7):370-372.

Chapter 4

Baroldi, G. et al. Sudden Coronary Death: A Postmortem Study in 208 Selected Cases Compared to 97 Control Subjects. *Am Heart Journal 1979*;98:20-31.
Brodsky, M. A. et al. Ventricular Tachyarrhythmia Associated with Psychological Stress. *JAMA* 1987;257:2064-2067.
Cannon, W. B. Voodoo Death. *Psychosomatic Medicine* 1957;19:182-190.
Eliot, R. S. *From Stress to Strength.* New York: Bantam Books, 1994.
Eliot, R. S. *Stress and the Heart-Mechanism, Measurement and Management.* New York: Futura Publishing, 1988.
Eliot, R. S., ed. *Stress and the Heart.* New York: Futura Publishing, 1974.
Engel, G. L. Death and Reunion: The Loss of a Twin. *Dartmouth Alumni Magazine* June 1981.
Engel, G. L. Sudden and Rapid Death During Psychological Stress, Folklore and Folk Wisdom. *Ann Intern Med* 1971;74:771-782.
Frankel, V. *Man's Search for Meaning.* New York: Simon & Schuster, 1959.
Goss, W. L. *The Soldier's Story.* Boston: Lee and Shepard, 1869.
Green, W. A, et al. Psychological Aspects of Sudden Death. *Arch Intern Med* 1972;129:775-73.
Lapin, B. A. and G. M. Cherkovich. Environmental Changes Causing the Development of Neuroses and Corticovisceral Pathology in Monkeys. In *Society, Stress and Disease: The Psychosocial Environment and Psychosomatic Diseases,* ed. L. Levi. London: Oxford University Press, 1971;1:266-279.

Lynch, J. et al. The Effects of Human Contact on Cardiac Arrhythmia in a Coronary Care Unit. *Journal of Nervous and Mental Disease* 1974;58:88-99.

Ruberman, W. et al. Psychosocial Influences on Mortality After Myocardial Infarction. *N Engl J Med* 1984;311:552-559.

Theil, H. G. et al. Stress Factors and Risk of Myocardial Infarction. *J Psychosomatic Res.* 1973;17:43-57.

Waller, B. F. and W. C. Roberts. Sudden Death While Running in Conditioned Runners Aged 40 and Over. *Am J Cardiology* 1980; 45(6); 1292.

Yawkes, M. L. Emotions as a Cause of Rapid and Sudden Death. *Archives of Neurology and Psychoanalysis* 1936;19:875-879.

Chapter 5

Alexander, F. W. *Psychosomatic Medicine: Its Principles and Applications.* New York: W. W. Norton and Co., 1950.

Anderson, K. M. et al. An Updated Coronary Risk Profile: A Statement for Health Professions. *Circulation.* 1991;83:356-32.

Bjorntorp, P. Regional Patterns of Fat Distribution. *Ann Int Med* 103; 1985:994-995.

Castelli, W. P. Cardiovascular Disease in Women. *Am J Obstet Gynecol* 1988;158:1153-1160.

Friedman, M. et al. Changes in the Serum Cholesterol and Blood Clotting Time in Men Subjected to Cyclic Variation of Occupational Stress. *Circulation* 1958;17:852-861.

Gey, G. F. et al. Inverse Correlation Between Plasma Vitamin E Consumption and Mortality from Ischemic Heart Disease in Crosscultural Epidemiology. *Am J Clin Nutr* 1991;53:326S-334S.

Gordon, T. and W. B. Kannel. Multiple Risk Functions or Predicting Coronary Heart Disease: The Concept, Accuracy, and Application. *Am Heart J* 1982;103:1031-1039.

Hertog, M. G. et al. Dietary Antioxidant Flavonoids and Risk of Coronary Heart Disease: The Zutphen Elderly Study. *Lancet* 1993;342:1007-11.

Joint National Committee on Detection, Evaluation, and Treatment of High Blood Pressure. The 1984 report of the Joint National Committee on Detection, Evaluation, and Treatment of High Blood Pressure. *Arch Intern Med* 1984;144:1045-1057.

Kannel, W. B. et al. A General Cardiovascular Risk Profile: The Framingham Study. *Am J Cardiol.* 1976;38:46-51.

Kannel, W. B. Update on The Role of Cigarette Smoking in Coronary Artery Disease. *Am Heart J.* 1981;101:319-328.

Kannel, W. B and P. Wilson. Risk Factors That Attenuate the Female Coronary Disease Advantage. *Arch Intern Med* 1995;155:57-61.

Kaplan, J. R. et al. Social Stress and Atherosclerosis in Normocholesterolemic Monkeys. *Science* 1983;220:733-735.

Kaplan, J. R. and S. B. Manuck. Stress-Induced Heart Rate Reactivity and Atherosclerosis in Monkeys. *Psychosom Med* 1981;43:189.

Keys, A., ed. Coronary Heart Disease in Seven Countries. *Circulation* Suppl. 1970;1 42:I-1-I-211.

Keys, A. Ten-Year Mortality in the Seven Countries Study. In: *Medical Aspects of Mortality Statistics*, H. Bostrom and N.. Ljungstedt, eds. The Skandia Group, Almqvist & Wiksell International, Stockholm, 1981.

Morris, D. L. et al. Serum Carotenoids and Coronary Heart Disease. *JAMA* 1994;272:1439-41.

Nerem, R. M. et al. Social Environment as a Factor in Diet Induced Aortic Atherosclerosis in Rabbits. *Science* 1980;208:1475-76.

Nixon P. Are There Clinically Significant Prodromal Signs and Symptoms of Impending Sudden Death? *Practical Cardiology*, 1982; 8:175-183.

Pickering, T. G. et al. Comparisons of Blood Pressure During Normal Daily Activities, Sleep, and Exercise in Normal and Hypertensive Subjects. *JAMA* 1982;247:992-996.

Renaud, S. and M. de Lorgeril. Wine, Alcohol, Platelets and the French Paradox for Coronary Heart Disease. *Lancet* 1992;339:1523-6.

Sinatra, S. T. and A. Lowen. Heartbreak and Heart Disease—The Origin and Essence of Coronary-Prone Behavior. *Holistic Medicine* 1987;2:169-172.

Sinatra, S. T. *Optimum Health* New York: Lincoln Bradley, 1996.

Taggert, P. and M. Carruthers. Endogenous Hyperlipidemia Induced by Emotional Stress of Racing Driving. *Lancet* 1971;1:16-22.

Ulbricht, T. L. and D. A. Southgate. Coronary Heart disease: Seven Dietary Factors. *Lancet* 1991;338:985-92.

Verschuren, W. M. M. et al. Serum Total Cholesterol and Long-Term Coronary Heart Disease Mortality in Different Cultures. *JAMA* 1995;274:131-136.

Chapter 6

Bly, R. *Iron John* New York: Vintage Books (Random House), 1992.

Lowen A. *Love, Sex and Your Heart.* Macmillan, 1988.

Sinatra, S. T. Heartbreak, Heartache, and Cardiac Pain—A Study of Coronary Prone Behavior. *Bioenergetic Analysis* 1987;1:55-63.

Sinatra, S. T. Aortic Dissection Associated with Anger, Suppressed Rage and Acute Emotional Stress. *J Cardiopulmonary Rehab* 1986;6:197-199.

Sinatra, S. T. and H. Hatch. Physiological and Psychological Profiles of Participants in a Six Day Healing the Heart Seminar. Unpublished data, 1987.

Tolkien, J. R. R. *The Lord of the Rings.* Boston: Houghton Mifflin Co., 1983 (1955).

Von Franz, M. L. *Shadow and Evil in Fairy Tales.* Dallas: Spring Publications Inc., 1987 (1974).
Woodman, M. *Addiction to Perfection.* Toronto: Inner City Books, 1982.

Chapter 7

Abramov, L. A. Sexual Life and Sexual Frigidity Among Women Developing Acute Myocardial Infarction. *Psychosomatic Medicine* 1976;38:418-424.
Achterberg, J. *Imagery and Healing: Shamanism and Modern Medicine.* Champaign, Ill.: Shambhala, 1985.
Achterberg, J. and F. Lawlis. *Imagery and Disease.* Institute for Personality and Ability Testing, 1984.
Benson, H. *The Relaxation Response.* New York: Avon Books, 1976.
Camaione, D. N. and S. T. Sinatra. Beneficial Effects of Exercise and Current Concepts in Adult Fitness. *Conn Medicine* 1981;45:620-624.
Cousins, N. *Anatomy of an Illness.* New York: W. W. Norton, 1979
Downing, G. *The Massage Book.* New York: Wildwood House, 1972.
Eliot, R. S, ed. *Stress and the Heart,* New York: Futura Publishing, 1974.
Greenberg, S. M. and W. H. Frishman. Co-Enzyme Q10: A New Drug for Cardiovascular Disease. *J Clin Pharmacol* 1990; 30:596-608.
Langsjoen, P. H. et al. Long-Term Efficacy and Safety of CoEnzyme Q10 Therapy for Idiopathic Dilated Cardiomyopathy. *Am J Cardiol* 1990;65: 512-523.
Lowen, A. *Bioenergetics.* New York: Penguin Books, 1976.
Lowen, A. *Fear of LIfe.* New York: Macmillan Publishing Company, 1980.
Lowen, A. and L. Lowen. *The Way to Vibrant Health: A Manual of Bioenergetic Exercises.* New York: Harper & Row, 1977.
Lowen, A. *Depression and the Body.* New York: Pelican Books, 1973.
Lowen, A. *Love and Orgasm.* New York: Macmillan Publishing Company, 1965.
Lowen, A. *Narcissism.* New York: Macmillan Publishing Company, 1984.
Lowen, A. *The Betrayal of the Body.* New York: Macmillan Publishing Company, 1967.
Lowen, A. *The Language of the Body.* New York: Macmillan Publishing Company, 1958.
Lynch, J. *The Broken Heart.* New York: Basic Books,1977.
Maresh, C. M. et al. Middle Age Male Distance Runners: Physiological and Psychological Profiles. *J Sports Med Phys Fitness* 1991;31:461-469.
McCully, K. S. Vascular Pathology of Homocysteinemia: Implications for the Pathogenesis of Arteriosclerosis. *Am J Pathol* 1969;56:111-128.
Michael, R. T. et al. *Sex in America: A Definitive Survey.* New York: Warner Books, 1995.

Mittleman, M. A. et al. Triggering of Acute Myocardial Infarction by Heavy Physical Exertion. *New Engl J of Medicine* 1993;329:1677-83.

Moriso, C. et al. Effect of Co-Enzyme Q10 Therapy in Patients with Congestive Heart Failure: A Long Term Multicenter Randomized Study. *Clin Invest* 1993;71:S134-S136.

Older, J. *Touching Is Healing.* New York: Stein and Day, 1982.

Ornstein, R. *The Healing Brain.* New York: Simon & Schuster, 1987.

Pierrakos, J. *Core Energetics.* Mendocino, Cal.: Life Rhythm Publishing, 1986.

Reich, W. *The Function of the Orgasm.* New York: Simon & Schuster, 1973.

Rider, M. S. et al. Effect of Immune System Imagery on Secretory IgA. *Biofeedback and Self-Regulation* 1990;15:317-333.

Sinatra, S. T. and J. DeMarco. Free Radicals, Oxidative Stress, Oxidized Low Density Lipoprotein (LDL), and the Heart: Antioxidants and Other Strategies to Limit Cardiovascular Damage. *Conn Medicine* 1995;59:579-588.

Sinatra, S. T. et al. Effects of Continuous Passive Motion, Walking, and a Placebo Intervention on Physical and Psychological Well-Being. *J Cardiopul Rehab* 1990;10:279-286.

Wabrek, A. J. and R. C. Burchell. Male Sexual Dysfunction Associated with Coronary Heart Disease. *Archives of Sexual Behavior* 1980;9:69-75.

Waller B. F. and W. C. Roberts. Sudden Death While Running in Conditioned Runners Aged 40 Years or Over. *Am J Cardiol* 1980;45(6):1292-1300.

Chapter 8

Elkind, D. *The Hurried Child.* Reading, Mass.: Addison-Wesley Publishing Co., 1981.

Lowen, A. *Narcissism.* New York: Macmillan Publishing Company, 1984.

Miller, A. *For Your Own Good.* New York: Noonday, 1983.

Miller, A. *Prisoners of Childhood.* New York: Noonday,1981.

Sinatra, S. T. and S. M. Hunter. Stress and Physiological Consequences to Youth. *Physician & Patient* April 1984: 23-28.

Chapter 9

Hafen, L. R. *Mountain Men and Fur Traders of the Far West.* Lincoln: University of Nebraska Press, 1982.

Harris, B. *John Colter.* Basin, Colo.: Big Horn Co., 1952.

Reich, W. *Character Analysis.* New York: Farrar, Straus & Giroux, 1945.

Sinatra, S. T. and H. Hatch. Physiological and Psychological Profiles of Participants in a Six Day Healing the Heart Seminar. Unpublished data, 1987.

Chapter 10

Buford, B. *Half Time.* Grand Rapids. Mich.: Zondervan Pub., 1994.

Byrd, R. C. Positive Therapeutic Effects of Intercessory Prayer in a Coronary Care Unit Population. *Southern Medical Journal* 1988; 81(7):826-29.

Collipp, P. The Efficacy of Prayer: A Triple Blind Study. *Medical Times* 1969;97.

Cortis B. *Heart and Soul.* New York: Villard Books, 1995.

Dossey, L. *Healing Words.* New York: HarperCollins, 1995.

Dreher, H. Boosting Heart Health with Spirit. *Natural Health,* March/April 1995.

Eddy, M. B. *Science and Health with Key to the Scriptures.* Boston: The First Church of Christ, Scientist, 1934.

Joyce, C. R. B. and R. M. C. Welldon. The Objective Efficacy of Prayer: A Double-Blind Clinical Trial. *J Chronic Disease 1965*;18:367-377.

Suggested Additional
Readings

————⟋————

Achterberg, J., B. Dossey et al. *Rituals of Healing: Using Imagery for Health and Wellness.* New York: Bantam Books, 1994.

Baker, E. F. *Man In The Trap.* New York: Collier Books, 1980.

Baumel, S. *Dealing with Depression Naturally.* New Canaan, Conn.: Keats Publishing, 1995.

Dyer, W. W. *Pulling Your Own Strings.* New York: Thomas Crowell, 1978.

Eliot, R. S. *Stress and Cardiovascular Diseases.* Armonk, New York: Futura Publishing, 1979.

Friedman, M. and D. Ulmer. *Treating Type A Behavior And Your Heart.* New York: Alfred A. Knopf, Inc., 1984.

Heagle, J. A. *Contemporary Meditation on Hope.* Chicago: Thomas More Press, 1975.

Jampolsky, G. G. *Love Is Letting Go of Fear.* Berkeley: Celestial Arts, 1979.

Keen, S. *Fire In The Belly: On Being a Man.* New York: Bantam Books, 1991.

Klatz, R., and R. Goldman. *Stopping the Clock.* New Canaan, Conn.: Keats Publishing, Inc., 1996.

Kubler-Ross, E. *To Live Until We Say Good-bye.* Englewood Cliffs, N.J.: Prentice-Hall, 1978.

Kushi, M. with A. Jack. *Diet for a Strong Heart.* New York: St. Martin's Press, 1985.

Laskow, L. *Healing with Love: A Physician's Breakthrough Mind/Body Medical Guide for Healing Yourself and Others.* San Francisco: HarperSanFrancisco, 1992.

Littarru, G. P. *Energy and Defense.* Italy: C.E.S.I., 1995.

Lowen, A. *Biogenergetics.* New York: Pelican Publishing Company, 1976.

Lowen, A. *Fear of Life.* New York: MacMillan Publishing Company, 1980.

Lowen, A. *Love, Sex and Your Heart.* New York: Macmillan Publishing Company, 1988, Penguin/Arcana Publishing Company, 1994.

Lowen, A. *Stress and Illness: A Bioenergetic View.* New York: 1980.

Lynch, J. J. *The Language of the Heart: The Human Body in Dialogue.* New York: Basic Books, 1985.

Meehan, B. *The Healing Power of Prayer.* Missouri: LiGuori, 1988.

Northrup, C. *Women's Bodies, Women's Wisdom.* New York: Bantam Books, 1994.

Ornstein, R. and C. Swencionis. *The Healing Brain: A Scientific Reader.* New York, Guilford Press, 1990.

Peck, M. S. *The Different Drum: Community Making and Peace.* New York: Simon and Schuster, Touchstone, 1987.

Rath, M. *Eradicating Heart Disease.* San Francisco: Health Now, 1993.

Siegel, B. S. *Peace, Love, and Healing.* New York: Harper & Row, 1989.

Simon, S. B. and S. Simon. *Forgiveness.* New York: Warner Books, Philip Lief Group, 1990.

Simonton, C. O., S. Matthews-Simonton and J. L. Creighton. *Getting Well Again: A Step-by-Step, Self-help Guide to Overcoming Cancer for Patients and Their Families.* New York: Bantam Books, 1978.

Sinetar, M. *Elegant Choices, Healing Choices.* New Jersey: Paulist Press, 1988.

Weil, A. *Spontaneous Healing.* New York: Alfred A. Knopf, Inc., 1995.

Widdowson, R. *The Joy of Yoga.* Garden City, N.Y.: Doubleday/Dolphin, 1983.

Williams, R. *The Trusting Heart: Great News About Type A Behavior.* New York: Times Books, 1989.

INDEX

251

About the Author

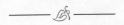

Stephen T. Sinatra, M.D. is a board-certified cardiologist and certified bioenergetic analyst with more than 10 years of post-graduate training in the crucial role behavior and emotion play in heart disease. For two decades, Dr. Sinatra has helped patients prevent and reverse heart disease utilizing conventional medical treatments as well as complementary nutritional and psychological therapies at his New England Heart Center in Manchester, Connecticut.

Dr. Sinatra is a fellow of the American College of Cardiology, Director of Medical Education at Manchester Memorial Hospital and an Assistant Clinical Professor of Medicine at the University of Connecticut School of Medicine. His articles have appeared widely in medical journals on traditional and alternative cardiology. The author of two previous books, *Lose to Win: A Cardiologist's Guide to Weight Loss* and *Optimum Health*, Dr. Sinatra serves as editor for *HeartSense*, a monthly newsletter devoted to healing the heart. Call 800-211-7643 for subscription information.